# Healing Hands

*By*

**Swami Nigmanand Sarasvati**

***Traditional Reiki Master***

**Books For All**

**Delhi**

*Published by*
**Books For All**
A-6, Nimri Commercial Centre,
Near Ashok Vihar Phase-IV,
Delhi-110052
Phones: 011-27302453, Fax: 011-47061936
e-mail: info@Lppindia.com
website: www.Lppindia.com

**Marketed By:**
**Low Price Publications**
A-6, Nimri Commercial Centre,
Near Ashok Vihar Phase-IV,
Delhi-110052
Phones: 011-27302453, Fax: 011-47061936
e-mail: info@Lppindia.com
website: www.Lppindia.com


First Published 2013
ISBN 10 : 81-7386-289-3
ISBN 13: 978-81-7386-289-2

*Printed at*
**D. K. Fine Art Press Pvt. Ltd.**
Delhi-110052



PRINTED IN INDIA

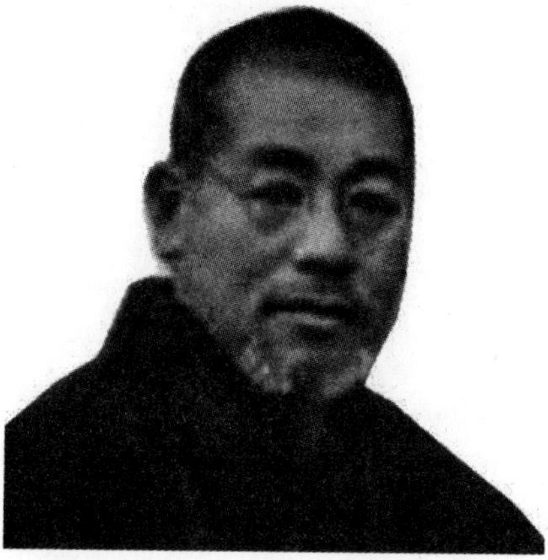

**Dr. Mikao Usui**
**Founder of Reiki-Healing**
**1864-1923**

Dedicated by the author to his
Reikei Master

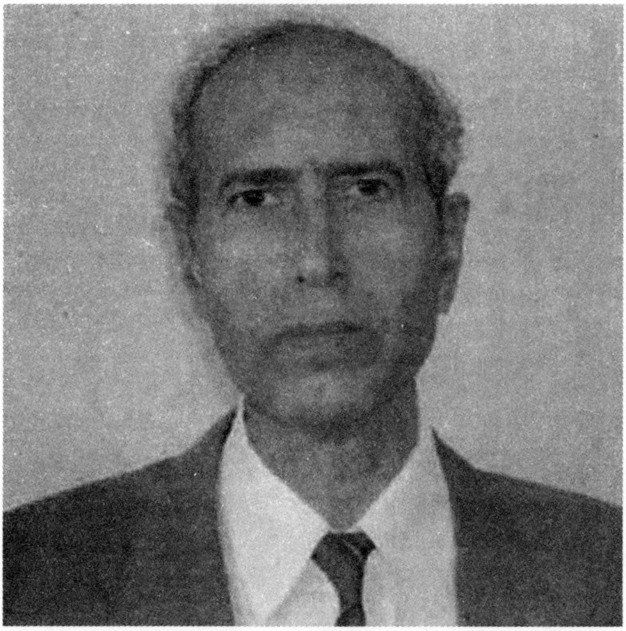

Shri Amarjit Oberoi,
New Delhi

# Contents

# Preface

This book gives comprehensive information about the health and spiritual practices. Usually books are overloaded with information and not focused at specifics. Reader finds it difficult to comprehend. However, I have tried to be simple and lucid in my presentation. The scope of Reiki is widened through the title as 'Healing Hands'.

There are several new topics enlisted in this book such as, Reiki signals, sixth principle, inviting the god of one's own fourth chakra, Buddha of the sixth chakra, Reiki on brain chambers, hempispheres, and chakras of the foot sole.

Interesting and new areas like mudras, clapping, balancing, Osho's meditations, sudarshan chakra, index finger, and see your aura, are also added. Nothing has been imagined and every aspect is on the basis of practical experience. I have also tried to provide a lot of useful information about the chakras.

The Author

# Invocation

Where there is Eternal Light,
Where there is Bliss,
In the safe and sound Eternity,
Place me there O! God.
Flow to me O! All Delight.

**Rig Veda 9-113-7**

Hail ! Celestial Light,
Shine inward and irradiate,
That I may see and tell,
Of things invisible to mortal sight
---------
Yet unattempted in prose or rhyme
--------
And fit audience find.

Paradise Lost Book- I
**- John Milton**

# 1. Spiritual Evolution

Why does a fish jump out of the sea? Because it wants to see what is beyond the sea? How is the life upon the earth? A fish out of water becomes restless and thinks that it has committed a mistake. It was happy in the sea. There was no need to come out. It may go back to the sea or die.

It may die or repent. It has a will to go further, to rise and grow. It will be given, by nature, the next birth in which it can live on earth or in the sea, as it wills. The birth will be in the form of a frog, tortoise, snake, cancer, crocodile and so on. Thus the physical evolution is preceded by spiritual evolution. The thought arises first and then the action takes place.

If you are poor and weak, try to be rich and healthy. If you are rich, serve the society, try to know what is beyond the body. If you are practicing yoga and meditations, search and experience more till you find whatever you want.

It is better to die for a noble cause.

In the poem, "Ulyses" written by Lord Alfred Tennyson, the king Ulyses at the age eighty says-

"How dull it is to pause, to make an end

To rust unburnished, not to shine in use

As though to breathe were life".

The desire for material progress ultimately turns into the will to grow spiritually in the process of evolution.

**My this hand is Abundant,**

**This one is even more.**

**My this hand is all medicines,**

**This one is touching the God.**

**Atharva Veda 4-13-6**

This mantra deals with three topics:

1. **Physical**- We can heal by the energy of touch.
2. **Psychological**- When the frequency of this energy increases, it creates abundance.
3. **Spiritual** - When the energy moves still beyond, the feeling of vastness and oneness leads to Divinity.

## 2. Physical Healing

According to Kirlian Photography, body of a healthy man emits light from all parts. If any part does not show light it will suffer from a disease after six months because it has lost the energy required to maintain it. If the light is regained subsequently, we can escape the disease. Light vanishes due to energy-blocks.Body becomes a bad conductor of energy.

# 3. Energy-Blocks

Suppressed energy of emotions like that of love, fear, jealousy hatred, anger, violence, worry, laughter, cry, sex, rigidity, dishonesty, cunningness, falsehood, resistance, competition, attachment, condemnation, lack of freedom, - is called an energy block. Blocks do not allow the waste energy to go out and fresh energy to come in. The part of the body loses light, becomes weak, we fall sick, depression is created and block is more fortified. Thus the man is entrapped in a vicious circle. These energy blocks are called Samskar, Karma Bandhanas, Granthies (knots), sanchit karmas in Sanskrit and Arman in Urdu language.

Gita says the worldly life is full of bondages. These are dreams, day - dreams, problems and dust on the mirror of soul. The dominant block is sent for action by sixth chakra, the other blocks can be dissolved by meditations.

These blocks stick to our body parts and are pictured in our aura– the vital or astral body (light through out the body) from toe to top.

The fire of suppressed emotions gives birth to the smoke of thoughts which cover our aura. Aura is a brilliant garment given by the God, but is stained by blocks. These blocks make our life feverish.

The world is too much with us,
Getting and spending we lay waste our powers,
Little we see in nature that is ours,
The malady is deeper hid,
The world is poisoned at the heart.

-William Wordsworth

# 4. Subconscious Mind

Group of these blocks of the whole body is called subconscious mind. It handles us like a robot. Its suppressed energy waves are always rising. It works when the conscious mind stops such as in dream or in the free time. It is called in Sanskrit Chanchalam Manah, the mind that walks too much. Thinking is its form of walking. We drain out more energy by seeing, hearing, speaking and thinking. This is why the deaf, dumb, blind and illiterate persons are stronger than the normal ones. Sub- conscious mind is like a broken mirror. We have to choose in which part to see our face. Our choice will not be ideal. Major block is desire and assumes all the forms of energy blocks.

We should work to fulfill the necessities of life and not the desires which are the causes of cycles of rebirth. The world is a reflection of our sub-conscious mind. We see and react accordingly.

# 5. Removal of Blocks

## (Polishing the mirror of Soul)

The suppression of emotions begins from childhood, becomes forceful in later age and causes diseases. 4th Chakra (middle of the chest) is the seat of love. It is psychological heart. Its gland is thymus. Its function is immunity. It fights with diseases. Hands are the motor organs and skin is the sense organ of 4th chakra. Love flows through hands and is received by the skin. Blocks are dissolved by touch. Divinity begins with the fourth chakra. So the touch though physical is the base of divinity.

If you are deprived of touch, touch yourself for an hour, on the whole body. Find out the part that dislikes touch, it is sick. Blocks are removed by touching, clapping, pressing, rubbing, striking, gazing, blowing, sweeping, massage and scratching. You can cut it into pieces by curved fingers, catch it like a ball and flick your hands. Negative energy of blocks is thick, it can be caught. When flicked, it is driven by the magnetic waves of the earth from North pole to South pole for purification. Do it daily. It is divine healing.

Blocks are removed by expressions directly or indirectly and completely by psychological treatment as is available in USA, mainly by laughter and crying. It is an advanced step of nature cure. No medicine is given.

Osho's meditations remove blocks and suppressed energy comes out. In my opinion such type of catharsis is not seen in Yoga and it is merely a poor physiotherapy.

Blocks are removed by Pranic healing and Reiki touch. Comparatively Reiki is the best, safe, practical, comfortable, complete, lasts life time & leading to the Ultimate. After removal of blocks, body becomes a good conductor of energy and we are cured of physical and mental diseases.In Sanskrit this condition is called Samadhi which is a state of ecstasy. Sama is taken from samadhan, the solution. Adhi means mental troubles like anger etc... Samadhi means the solution of the mental troubles which are root causes of diseases.

## 6. Necessity of Loving Touch

So, touch is a necessity, even animals do like touch. A child receives touch in his mother's womb from all sides. Even after birth, the children who are deprived of touch often die. Those who survive acquire negative tendencies. Those who do not receive the touch of their family, receive the professional touch of doctors and nurses but it is too late. The diseased part of our body dislikes touch. In Liverpool University scientists have discovered that the soft and gentle touch activates pleasure nerves and thus relieves pains.

All our knowledge is based on touch. We gain knowledge by touch of eyes, ears, tongue, nose and skin. Touch is a form of love and love is a form of diet. When the child is fed from mother's breast it gets both love and diet and diet is therefore identified with love. Children who are deprived of love eat more and those who are loved more eat comparatively less and same is the case with elderly persons.

## 7. History of Touch

Due to social changes, Vedic culture did not remain popular and was confined to a few persons. A part of this culture is seen in Padama (Lotus) sutra of Lord Buddha and in the Bible - 'Curing through energy by hands'. In Japan Mr. Mikao Usui, Dean of the Christian Academy, devoted his whole life to find out the truth. He travelled in all the European countries, studied Buddhist literature, Vedas and concluded that it is possible, if one is enjoined with the universal energy.

He observed fast for 21 days, practiced all the meditations he knew, and on the last day he saw a current of bright light with 4 symbols entering his head. His body vibrated with energy. His hands became healing hands and he founded Reiki, the art of natural healing. He cured and taught Reiki to so many persons in Japan. His follower lady Takata taught Reiki in USA and there after this learning spread throughtout the World.

# 8. Pranic Energy- Reiki

**"Sun is rising as the Prana of all Creatures", - Veda.**

Pranic energy is not original. It is a radiation of Sun, Moon, Earth stars, diamonds, stones, metals, trees, animals, creatures and so on. It is fluctuating and not found equally everywhere, at all times. It is found more in the morning, in greenery and lonely places, and less in the night, in cities, crowded places and desert. Less means, less positive and more negative.

The total amount of energy in the universe is always the same. It is bi-polar, like the rose plant with thorns and flowers or lotus in the mud. Its opposite is rayee in Upnishad and apana in yoga. Sun is prana, a positive current and moon is rayee the negative current. These two currents of energy create bi-polar objects. Pranic energy is only for physical healing and should be used carefully to avoid the negative energy of the patient. Master Choa Kok Sui in Philippines (Manilla) is its the founder. It is akin to nature cure.

Prana is thinner than negative energy but thicker than Reiki As per Indian mythology Reiki can be called Brahma. Word prana is frequently used in India, and therefore it seems supreme. Prana is a lower energy than Reiki and is its by-product.

## Reiki

**"Purusha is all, whatever has happened and will happen"**
– Rig Veda

Purusha is the Universal Man. It is the energy in all forms and activities of the world. He is said to be of fair colour and else where called Brahman. In quantum physics Albert Einstein first gave the idea that the matter and energy is one and the same thing. Matter is freezed energy ($e=mc^2$) Energy is everything.

In Japanese Language Rei means universal and Kei means energy. So Reiki means Universal energy. It is the origin of universe and everything in it. In all things only the frequency differs. Solid things have low frequency and all others have high frequency. Our body, thoughts and the emotions are all its forms.

Frequency of sleep is low, of meditation high and of Moksha the highest. Sankhya philosophy says–these are all the forms of Brahma.

It is all pervading, and of white colour, found equally every where at all times. It is one and non-polar, hence balancing and transcending dualities. It has intelligence, awareness, wonder, love, peace, grace, bliss and further deep-detachment. That detached form is believed as God. This energy is original.

# 9. Reiki Initiations

In Vajra Yana sect of Buddhism, initiation is in its real sense. In Veda, Vajra means the weapon of Lord Indra, the king of gods, Literally the vajra means a stone. Lightning is his weapon. During rains when lightning takes place germs are killed on the earth and in the atmosphere if there are rains without lightening germs grow and germicides are used. Yana means ship, here it means a sect. Lightning shows also the way to the traveller at night.

In initiation, the Reiki master draws symbols on the chakras, the energy wheels of our body and we begin to get energy from the universe. Every cell of our body is lit up and it keeps us healthy and shows the way to grow spiritually. Initiation once taken is sufficient forever. However extra initiations are beneficial. After initiation, student becomes a Reiki Channel. It is an important event in life. Student sees light, visions, feels light or heaviness, heat during irritation depending on his body - frequency. Some do not have any experience. They should take more initiations to enhance the frequency of the body. Initiation should be validated by practice and experience.

There are three degrees of initiations. Energy increases gradually in these degrees. First degree deals with physical, second with mental and distant healing and the third with spiritual healing. In Sanskrit it is called Shaktipat, showering of energy.

# 10. Energy Exchange

It is an eternal law of nature that energy exchange, maintains the universal movement, creates a balance and fortifies the relations. It unburdens both the giver and the receiver.

Otherwise, the burden creates an energy block. It shows the sense of gratitude, activates the 6$^{th}$ chakra, the master chakra and its gland-pituitary. Scientists have observed that there is a process of exchange even in the tiniest part of the matter like electrons. There is a beauty of behavior and satisfaction in exchange.

When somebody works for us or given us something, in exchange, we should pay him for his work. Now a days money is a superior means of exchange. Therefore, you must pay the fee to the Reiki Master for the initiation or healing received.

German Reiki master Walter Luback proposes 'Fair Offering' instead of paying fee. We become related to the Reiki Master for the whole life. Relation should be based on love, pay him respectfully before hand whatever you can and you will get whatever you deserve. If we pay the fee after the initiation it is a temporary business and not the love.

One who breaks the law of exchange, he will lose in the long run. Nature will some day make him pay back fully as every thing is recorded in sub-conscious mind. One who does not want to pay has closed the doors for the entry to Reiki and will not gain anything.

If a Reiki student is actually not in a position to pay fee, Reiki master should give him some money to pay back as his fee. This is also sufficient to maintain the law. If a Reiki master does not want to take fee, he is an egoist and will suffer one day. And one who does not want to give, will be some day reduced to a pauper. You may help any person without showing your ego.

Exchange is a sense of return. Clouds are formed by sea water. Clouds rain. Rivers flow towards the sea. Life on the earth is thus maintained.

Reiki can be given to a person as a gift. If you don't find any person for Reiki, return the energy to the universe.

Balancing is all. When energies are totally balanced,we achieve peace, love, Moksha. Energy exchange is a main feature in balancing our activities of life. Energy exchange is a cross-ventilation which keeps us healthy. It is another form of earning and spending. Both are necessary to maintain personal and social life.

# 11. Inviting Reiki and Five Principles

Keep your hands and mind in a prayerful mood.

i. I thank (Name) as a healer for being here.

ii. I thank Reiki for being here.

iii. I thank (Name) as healee for being here.

iv. I thank Master Mikao Usui for being here.

v. I thank my Reiki master (Name) for being here.

vi. I thank gods and spiritual guides for being here

vii. I thank the god of my fourth chakra and Lord Buddha of my sixth Chakra for being here.

Call compels an answer. Watch the flow of energy in your hands

I. **Five Principles of Reiki -**

I obey the principles of Reiki.

i. I will live honestly today.

ii. I will not worry today.

iii. I will not be angry today.

iv. I will love and respect everybody today.

v. I will be grateful to everybody today.

vi. Self added principle - I will maintain balance in my life today.

**Affirmation**

1. I accept divine order.
2. I am an instrument of Reiki. I am getting Love, Peace, Grace, Intelligence, Blessings and energy of Reiki in abundance along with the other persons of Reiki.
3. I desire good for all.

This invocation can be used as daily prayer by every body. Invocation is sufficient once or twice a day. On other times you can go without it, because energy moves by intention alone. Hands on, Reiki on; Hands off, Reiki off.

## 12. Method of Healing, First Degree

After invocation wait and watch the flow of energy in your hands. See that Reiki is flowing from seventh chakra (Crown) from your head to $4^{th}$, the heart chakra and thence to the hands.

Now put your hands in a spoon shape on the part of the body and say "I am being healed at (name of the part)". Touch of both hands or at least one hand should be maintained by slipping from one part of the body to another through out the healing process. Wear loose cotton clothes and as less as required. Though Reiki goes to the body even if you keep a distance of one inch but direct touch is more useful for knowing the feelings, keep fingers touching each other, not scattered, finger tips of both hands should not touch each other. Touch softly, do not press.

# 13. Parts of Body

Main seven chakras, their glands,organs and joints.

1. One hand on crown chakra and one stretched with palm upwards
2. Temples
3. Sixth chakra - between eyebrows and back of head.
4. Hemispheres
5. Brain chambers - back, middle and front head - two parts each
6. Eyes
7. Ears
8. Throat pit and back
9. Thymus and middle chest - fourth chakra
10. Lungs
11. Shoulders (end of the collar bone upper pit)
12. Navel
13. Liver
14. Spleen
15. Hara (below navel) $2^{nd}$ chakra
16. Thigh Joints
17. Root Chakra

18. Knees (below knee bone)
19. Foot sole
20. Yang - Yin chakra. (Right + left below shoulder chakras)
21. Elbows
22. Wrists
23. 4th chakra back
24. Navel back
25. Kidneys - back
26. Hara back - tail of the back bone

At the end say - Thank you Reiki, I am healed.

There are seven chakras in the foot sole. Those belong to our past animal life. Those chakras also need initiation and Reiki. In Vedic ritual (yajna) parts of body are touched hurriedly within two minutes with fingers dipped in water, and Prayer is made to God to make those parts strong. These are the remains of Reiki healing.

Draw Reiki for three minutes on each part, one minute for children, thirty minutes extra should be given to the diseased parts.

Always move hands from head to feet, from top to bottom to flush down the negative energy to the earth. No part of body is taboo. Every part of body is a potential Reiki position.

To save time draw Reiki on the hemispheres, chakras of the body and foot sole. For the back parts, a partner is required. Husband and wife can be good partners for each other. Don't cross legs during Reiki practice.

## 14. Benefits of Reiki

Unlike pranic energy, it is always fresh and abundant. In second degree you can also give or receive Reiki from a distant place. One who gives Reiki to any body he himself gains because Reiki also flows through his body and therefore, he should be happy. We can heal the dead, the past and future events and relationships. There is psychic surgery also. We can call the gods. We can not harm any body even by conscious or unconscious effort, unlike the black magic. We can grow spiritually to the utmost limit. In Reiki healing you get the energy from out side, you can get it in abundance. You do not require any diet or medicine.

## 15. Feelings of Reiki Healing

1. On some parts of the body you will feel heat, pain, numbness or irritation.This means the block is melting and negative energy flowing out. Catch it like a ball and flick your hands. Give Reiki again. Here you will feel your palm being pushed upward.
2. Some times we feel that palm is being sucked and pulled down. It means the part is receiving energy.
3. Some times you will feel light, it means the part is healthy and has more energy. It leads to oneness, awareness, and the feeling of vastness. It is the spiritual use of hands.
4. When Reiki stops, sensation in palm ends. Proceed further.
5. If Reiki is flowing but the part is not being healed, it means Reiki is going to another important part where it is most needed.
6. If the patient is wrecked too much or is about to die, Reiki will not flow.
7. Reiki flows through the giver and therefore, he is also benefitted. While giving the initiations, Paula Horan experienced that she was sharing the initiations.
8. While giving Reiki to somebody, synchronize your breath with his breath. Breath in and breath out along with him to know his feelings. When the blocks are scattered, Reiki resounds. If you give Reiki on the points of foot sole, it goes to the upper parts of the body and vice versa . It means the smooth flow of energy has taken place. Then single part treatment (only of seventh chakra) will do.

# 16. Reiki Signals

Reiki guides life through symbolical images. We should be able to read between the lines. During Reiki, after second degree initiation, the power increases and guidance begins on the subject, we are concerned. Images are attended by intuitive thoughts so do not think but listen. Sometimes the meaning is realized after four or five hours or days.

I had written a paper on Balancing Energies and wanted somebody to confirm the same. During my Reiki practice I saw a sieve. Again after 2 or 3 days I saw fine particles were sieved and the rough particles remained on the sieve. It means balancing is the crux of all yoga and meditations. Be Confident.

Then twice I saw a burning match stick, as we burn the match stick for lighting fire and preparing food. Health, wealth and meditations start all with the law of balancing. While giving Reiki on second chakra (of water supply) I saw mud which, to me, meant cleanse by devoting more time. After doing so I saw ice, white color, moon and mirror which meant clear. During the period of my mudra study and practice I saw my left hand upward, fingers scattered and thumb caught by the fingers of right hand. After thinking for long, I concluded that this is the suitable mudra for me although it is not found any where in the books. So I named it Arun Mudra. It flows the current of energy to the heart through the thumb, which is good for heart diseases.

The persons who invented something in dreams it was by the Reiki signals, like the structure of the carbon invented by Kequal.

He saw serpents holding each other's tail in their mouth in square shape. That was a symbol. Master Mikao Usui saw four symbols. Those were Reiki signals for him. Scripts of all languages are Reiki signals.

## 17. Second Degree -Mental and Distance Healing

Necessities of life such as air, water, grains and ground are easily available and given in abundance by nature. If any body suffers, it is due to mal-distribution in the society. Precious items are rarely found. Everybody cannot get those rare items and should not desire to get them. But a common man desires material and luxurious abundance.

It is said in a yoga book - "man gets all types of gems when he is deeply established in the feelings of non-stealing" Name of the third chakra is Manipur, it means the city of gems. It denotes that when the third chakra is fully activated man lives like a king in the city of gems.

Similarly people think that Kuber mudra makes a man rich. Every year on the night of Diwali festival, Laxmi, the goddess of wealth is worshiped with a hope of being rich. Reiki students also think that they can be rich by positive affirmation for money with the practice of Reiki.

As per Paula Horan's book "Abundance Through Reiki" Reiki gives only the sense of abundance and not material abundance. Therefore it is essential to express the emotion of abundance in inviting Reiki.

Even by getting abundant wealth, the cause of happiness is the sense of abundance, not the abundance itself. Sense of abundance is a wealth of satisfaction. Kabir says when a man gets the wealth of satisfaction, gold loses it glitter and diamonds their glow. It follows the gems seen in the meditations.

Abundance means limitless, feeling of vastness, without thoughts and desires but bliss, peace, delight, oneness, awareness, emptiness, silence, truth, eternal law (Dharma), infinity, eternity. All dualities end here. Both are balanced and transcended. This is the multiple experience of all the people in the world. All beauty, ugliness goodness, evils and errors equally contribute to the wealth of the Absoute. It is a hidden harmony in the universe.

The emptiness is positive, it is the origin of the world. So it is wholeness, fullness. This is called Bhooma in Upanishad - all - happiness. Limitation (Alpa) is sorrow. Urdu poet Mirza Galib says a drop of water when dropped in ocean enjoys abundance. Even the pain when exceeds its limit becomes medicine in itself. We get all, by losing all. This is a divine gambling, a paradox. We want to be happy by fulfilment. We can achieve it by emptiness. In Upanishad it is said, that such a person enjoys all types of happiness with God.

In second and third degrees the symbols, the method and the literature is provided by the Reiki master. If a student practises Reiki by drawing symbols for three years then his chakras are opened. Flow of Reiki in his body becomes very smooth and his healing power increases.

Bliss can be experienced after awaking from sound sleep. Sound sleep is possible if we are balanced and thoughtless at that time. Sleep is a transcendance. These days people have lost their sleep which can be achieved by Reiki. By the initiation of second degree the frequency of our power increases and body becomes a good conductor of energy.

**An Experience:**

Lie down with free mind and relax the body. Put your hands on thigh joints. Invoke and begin Reiki for one hour. Your hands are subject and your thigh joints are objects of feeling. With a good practice of a few days you will realize that your hands and thigh joints melt . These are so much filled with energy that you do not feel physical presence of hands and thigh joints. You have even forgotten your body. You feel one energy only. Feeling of duality - the subject - object sense is transcended. This is abundance, vastness and emptiness. Every thing originates from and dissolves in it. This state of abundance is called Eeshvar in Hindu religion.It is a road less traveled and some one has also written a book named, **"The Road Less Traveled".**

## 18. Third Degree - Spiritual Healing

In first degree Reiki we feel the physical touch. In second degree we feel the touch of energy sent from a distant place. Further we feel oneness and meet with intelligence, wonder, love, peace, bliss, grace and ultimately the detachment. All these are the fine forms of energy. There is no touch because duality is left behind. There is only an experience beyond and the beyond. Frequency of energy increases by practice. God can not be touched physically, it is only an awareness.

To grow spiritually one should have a broad outlook about religion. Those who think that their religion is supreme in the world, cannot rise. The ultimate attachment with the Guru (Master) is a hindrance. Master is a door to the journey of loneliness and not a wall to check you. You must respect the master even after enlightenment but have your own confidence to live and decide alone. Disciples of Lord Buddha and Mahaveer were enlightened when their masters left the body because attachment became a detachment on that moment.

# 19. Yoga Anatomy

## Chakras (Introduction)

**"Vehicle of human body has seven wheels pulled by seven horses"**

- Veda.

In Sanskrit Chakra means a wheel. These are energy centres where energy moves like a wheel. The chakras are in the back bone. If activated these get energy from the universe. There are mainly seven chakras. Some people think that chakras are fictitious. Hirsohi Motoyama, doctor of Acu - punture in Japan has made a machine which shows the working of chakras.

1. **Root chakra (Mooladhar)** it is in the perineum, between anus and testicles. In Reiki, energy goes to it through thigh - joints. Its motor organ is anus, sense organ is nose, its element is earth and essence is smell. It creates bone - structure of the body and whatever is solid in it. It gets energy from earth and Saturn. It vibrates in the crowd. Its energy is apan opposite of prana. It struggles for survival and sanity. Its glands are adrenals.

2. **Svadhishathana** (self abode) -Sacral or spleen chakra and Hara in Japanese. Animal life ends in root chakra and human life begins. On root chakra man also lives like animal. Psychologically human life begins from second chakra.

   This chakra is at the bottom of the back bone. Its front part is abdomen - below the navel. It circulates water in the body and changes into fluids. Its element is water, quality is taste. Its motor organs are kidneys, spleen, urinary organ and sense organ is tongue. It takes energy from the rays of moon. Its gland is gonad, i.e., testicles in males and ovaries in females.

3. **Navel Chakra**- Back side of navel. Its function is digestion. Its motor organ is liver, its gland is pancreas. Its sense organs are eyes and it receives energy from the sun. It is called Manipur in Sanskrit. It gives us the ability to social education and desire for fame and leadership. It is the tree of knowledge. Its fruit is forbidden. Its element is fire, its essence is appearance, its energy is sama - means equal - it equally distributes energy to all organs. If it is weak, it creates anger and violence.

4. **Anahata Chakra** - Anahata means unstruck sound. There is a self produced humming sound akin to soham (I am that - God).This chakra is the seat of love. Its star is Venus. Its motor organs are hands and sense organ is skin. Its element is air, quality is touch. Its energy is prana. It is located behind the middle of chest in the back. Its gland is thymus and function is immunity. Its weakness causes fatness and lack of love.

5. **Throat Chakra** - located in the neck, its gland is thyroid, its function is speech (communication). Its motor organ is tongue, sense organs are ears. Its element is space, quality is word. It works for purity, and turns poison into nectar and vice versa if weak. Its power is udan. Its star is mercury.

6. **Ajna Chakra** - Ajna means order - This chakra is a master chakra also called Guru. Its gland is pituitary - the master gland - Red in colour and located in the middle head. The chakra is in the back side of eye brows. It regulates all chakras and maintains the balance in the body. It is beyond 5 elements. Its star is Jupiter. It is called $6^{th}$ sense. Sub - conscious mind is its sense organ, hemispheres are its motor organs It is also called mind - chakra.

7. **Seventh Chakra** - It is located at the back of middle head where Hindus keep hair - tuft. Its gland is peneal. It is called

crown chakra, in Sanskrit called Sahasrar - means thousand petalled flower.

Thousands of energy rays come from universe and join here and looks like a multi colored flower. It is just opposite to Root chakra. The root chakra makes body solid like statue and seventh chakra's rays melt the body into a spiritual being, makes it invisible. Seventh chakra is the chakra of complete freedom.

In The Bible the chakras are called staircase of Heaven. Heaven begins from fourth chakra.

**"Seek ye first the kingdom of heaven and all other things shall be added unto thee". - Bible**

First and seventh chakra have no areas as others. These chakras receive and emit energy by themselves.

Chakras move anti clokwise and up and down when they receive energy and circulate it to the upper and lower chakras. When they project negative energy of the body they move clockwise in their fixed places. The first is positive and the second is negative charge.

**Channels**

According to Tantra books there are 72 thousand energy channels in the human body connected with chakras and organs. These channels receive energy from chakras and supply to the body parts. These are not blood vessels but ethereal and can be photographed by high frequency camera. Amongst these the following three channels are important.

**1. Pingla 2. Ida 3. Sushumana**

All these begin from root chakra. Pingla and ida go up to 6th chakra touching each chakra in a serpentine way. Pingla is of red color, ida of yellow and sushumana of white.(Reiki)

1. **Pingla** employs us in physical activity, material pleasures, logic and struggle. Its organ is liver. It is a solar energy. It is connected with left hemisphere of the brain and when it works our right

side is active. This can be known by the breathing of right side of nose and can be thus controlled. It has a mechanical property, because it activates our motor organs. Its working is positive charge.

2. **Ida** gives us rest, creative pleasures like music or poetry and fine arts. Its knowledge is intuitive. It is connected with the left side of the body and with the right hemisphere of the brain, it can be known and controlled by left side breathing of nose. It activates and keeps the left side of the body healthy. It is lunar. Its organ is spleen. It controls the sense organs of the body. Its working is negative charge.

3. **Sushumana** - when both ida and pingla are balanced the third channel sushumana becomes active. It contains and controls both the channles and gives awareness. First two channels end in 6$^{th}$ chakra. These keep us in worldly activity. Sushumana gives us awareness and leads to vastness and oneness. After 6$^{th}$ chakra ida stops and pingla as a vehicle, goes with sushumana. It leads us in the middle and front head, universal and personal awareness. When we are traveling in a train we are active and restful both. Such is the function of sushumana. As there is an earth - point in the plug, so sushumana is space - point in the bio - electricity. It is neutral.

It contains the qualities of joy and sorrow. Here seriousness becomes serenity. Working of sushumana can be known by the equal and simultaneous breathing by both nostrils. Breath becomes so soft and thin that it seems almost nil. Pingla digests solid food, ida liquid, and sushumana needs no food. So there is no desire for eating and drinking, or anything else. There are some people who do not take anything for days and months together.

**Aura**

**"It is not the eyes or nose or lips we beauty call,**

**But the total and joint impression of all".**

**- Alexander Pope**

**"She walks in beauty"**

**- Lord Byron**

There is something around our body. Matter has an etheric charge (ionized gas, plasma) around it. In living beings it is called aura in Latin, bio-plasma in Russian and Tejas in Sanskrit language. This is energy field scattered by our chakras. This is also called vital force or astral body. Animals and trees also have their aura. It is about one inch in side our body (as chakras are) and about two inches out side. It is called inner aura. In a healthy man its rays are spread up to three feet. Those are called health rays or outer aura. It is our shadow even in the darkness. Commonly it is called soul which has non-physical presence. Some people have written books on "Body Electronics".and "Human Astomphere" about the aura. There are 4 layers of aura around our body. As per Upnishad, it is concluded that there are five auras within the body. First aura is not the aura but is physical body. To some people the group of energy channels gives a feeling of aura within our body. The developed auras are like the spread out feathers of a dancing peacock.

1. **The Vital Aura**- It is called Pranamaya Kosh in sanskrit. It is formed by the energy rays of first and second chakra. Vital aura is yellow in colour and develops around the Trees, animals and illiterates.

2. **Mental Aura** - called Manomaya Kosh in Sanskrit. It is formed by 3rd chakra and is red in colour. It enables us to receive the education given by the society and to think about past and future. One can notice the difference between the educated and illiterate persons, both have different personality and act differently.

3. **Emotional Aura (Vignanmaya Kosh) -**

   (Here vignan does not mean science). It is formed by 4th chakra. As love is the seat of 4th chakra, this aura is developed by love added by meditations and is green in colour. This can extend to the aura of the earth, as our speed increases in the train during traveling.Here astral traveling is possible. Then one can say soham - “I am That”. The persons who glide in the air with the help of a parachute or a glider within the core of their heart they have the desire for astral traveling. Some of them die. Meditations of fourth chakra are required for their survival. Eienstein imagined the journey at the speed of light. It will be possible by astral traveling.

4. **Cosmic Aura (Anandamaya kosh)** - when one realizes awareness, endlessness, bliss and delight he identifies himself with the universal aura. It is formed by the sixth chakra, and is in dark blue colour. Body becomes super conductor of universal energy. Universal aura is called Hiranaya Garbh in Sanskrit.

**Halo** - In sanskrit it is called Ojas. When the rays of energy extend up to 6 inches on the 7th chakra, the grandeur is called halo. Crowns are poor replica of the halo. These auras can be photographed by Kirlian photography. In every activity of life be conscious of your aura throughout the day. You will feel delighted and dignified in your actions.

Aura goes out of the body in the dream, and gets connected with the dominent chakra and comes back through it. Be aware when you wake up out of a horror dream, you will see something entering your body and that is returning of aura. Scanning and sweeping of aura is essential in pranic healing but optional in Reiki because Reiki is an intelligent energy and flows to other parts of body when overdosed. Pranic energy is not loving and intelligent, works like a machine and makes a pranic congestion. There are chakras, channels and auras in every cell of our body. This is a grand design.

# Appendix

More lights on previous topics.and some new topics are added.

1. See your aura
2. Suppressed emotions.
3. Removal of blocks -
4. Five principles
5. Parts of body
6. Tree of Human body
7. Pranic energy.
8. Sea salt
9. Positive affirmations.
10. Clapping
11. Mudras
12. Index finger
13. Sudarshan chakra
14. More about chakras
15. Imagination of colours
16. Yoga postures
17. Enlightenment & Brain chambers
18. Balancing Energies
19. Emptiness

20. White light imagination
21. Dragon Breath
22. Controlling Mind
23. Desires
24. Company of Angels
25. Evolution
26. Dark Energy
27. Healing
28. Reiki Master
29. Sub-concious mind

**See Your Aura by Gazing in the Mirror**

Gazing in the mirror is useful for balancing and knowing the aura. It makes breath very soft and thin. In the beginning of meditation it arouses fear.

**Method** - Sit before a big mirror in which you can see half of your upper body. Make the room dark, light a lamp beside the mirror, so that it does not get reflected.No articles should get reflected from the mirror. If you wear spectacles do not remove them. See the image of each eye separately in front of it. If you have difficulty, gaze at the nose tip and then gaze at the eyes again. At times you will be successful but sometimes you will see images of both eyes with one eye. This is imbalance and remains through out your life. When you are balanced, you will see that the image of your face is washed off and the mirror does not reflect.

You will feel fog in the room and be connected with the energy having lost grip of matter. After one hour or when you end the meditation, you will see a yellow strip of light around your body, that is your vital aura.

This method is easily available and beneficial. Kirlian photography is costly and not available in every place. After being photographed your aura may change due to depression and mishappening.

Practise it for 90 days, twice daily, one hour at a time in the night, and early morning.

**2. Know your aura**- choose a big ground. Run as fast as you can and stop suddenly. You will see that someone is still running and that is your astral body, your aura. Aura expands in joy, peace, freedom and meditations. It shrinks and breaks by fear, sadness and bondage.

**Suppressed Emotions**

Some times we get very angry over trifle issues and let out our suppressed emotions. At times we let out our hidden emotions with laughter, crying and greed.

**Places of Suppression in Body**

1. Sex is blocked in root chakra in the form of fever and is passed on from one generation to another. This can be eradicated forever by Reiki healing. Intensity of sex, anger and the temperature in fever is one and the same. Do not draw Reiki on root chakra during fever else temperature will increase. Draw on second chakra for sweating.
2. Fear blocks the knees resulting in pain.
3. Greed, worries, laughter and crying block second chakra, stop excretion, create constipation and cause urinary diseases.
4. Ego, anger and violence block third chakra, resulting in impaired digestion, H.BP & L.BP, fatal diseases and accidents.
5. Grief (lack of love - while giving and receiving) blocks fourth chakra and creates heart and lung diseases.
6. Falsehood and Lack of gratitude block fifth chakra and cause diseases of throat.
7. Rigidity blocks sixth chakra, causes brain diseases and lack of intuition.

8. Irresponsibility or over responsibility blocks shoulder chakras.
9. Jealousy blocks small chakra near the physical heart.

**Exposure**

Daily keep your Reiki hand on the navel for as much time as you can. After some days you will feel heat and irritation, due to suppressed anger. Hold it like a ball and flick it off. After a few days you will feel comfort and relieved.

**Removal of Blocks by Activating Sixth Chakra**

Third chakra is the master of conscious mind. It determines our outward behavior and actions. If it is weak, the efficiency of our work and speech will be less.

Sixth chakra is the master of the sub-conscious mind. If it is normal, we control our emotions and if weak, we burst out. Anger is temporary. If we are too weak we become mad.

Women and children have less blocks than men because of their less resistance. Blocks are in the form of layers one over the other and heaps upon the heaps. These blocks are of joy and sorrow. When one block is exhausted the next beneath comes over, till all the blocks are exhausted. Blocks go up to fifth chakra. As the man evolves from one chakra to another the nature of blocks changes. Blocks are dominated by the upper chakras.

In Geeta Lord krishna says "One whose deeds are burnt in the fire of knowledge, is called a pandit". We receive knowledge imposed by society, which is laboriously built memory. It makes body weak and projects ego. This knowledge is gained by third chakra.

Knowledge of sixth chakra is intuitive,it is illumination, revelation, spontaneous, and right. Burning of deeds means ending all the energy blocks. As in the military parade, all the soldiers act as per order of the commander. Sixth chakra may use the blocks to relive past life. If desirable, it may dissolve those at once. It is a chakra of will power, can dismiss all the blocks and enable us to enter emptiness.

**Removal of Blocks** - (Osho) upasana meditation. Upasana means sit within yourself. People perform rituals in upasana while their mind wanders else where.

**Method** - Close the room and sit comfortably, watch your thoughts and emotions rising in the mind. Do what you want. If no emotion rises sit or lie down silently. After two or three days when your energy level goes up, you will feel emotions coming out. We are conditioned from the very childhood, as how to sit, lie down or stand. We do not do otherwise. Do as you like. The energy held there will get released and the block will melt. This is physical upasana.

**Oral** - speak what you like, without thinking whether it is good or bad. Sigmond Freud told his patients to speak what they wanted without any hitch. Patients got relieved and felt light at heart.

**Dancing** - Dance by the inner instincts without any planning for 40 minutes. In this case, all the stored energy blocks will get released and you will feel light. Lie down for 20 minutes for complete deconditioning of the body and mind. Meerabai was enlightened by dancing. The memory keeps working and one cannot get rid of thoughts and enter awareness while dancing after learning professional dancing.

Stars look like dancing in the universe and so are all the particles of our body. By suppressing the desire to dance we have become a robot and are cut off from universal energy. Dance develops aura of fourth chakra, and sometimes we come out of the body and see our selves. Russian dancer Nijinsky always saw himself dancing. Aura controls our body as a robot by will. Such persons can attend their own funeral like the Arch Bishop Haslam in the works of Bernard Shaw.

**Celebration and Entertainment**

Dancing, playing or singing is a celebration. It gives us full satisfaction and clears all the energy blocks. We grow spiritually and enjoy peace.

Due to social fear we cannot celebrate but can only see certain actions.

Seeing is a poor consolation which creates a new energy block and we intend to see more and more. People waste their time in seeing games, films and serials all the day. Those who perform the shows know the psychology of the persons seeing and earn money and fame.

## Five Principles

Mere recitation of five principles every day will not bring progress in life. You have to accept your weaknesses. Dishonesty, worries, anger, violence, lack of love, truth, respect and gratitude are due to the weakness of chakras.

Draw as much Reiki on chakras as you can. Undergo psychological treatment for avoiding anger and worries etc. Laughter in the morning and weeping in the evening are the cleansing processes. Have patience to get rid of these Mere observations of these emotions will do, as observation is the function of 6th chakra. It transforms energy and raises it upward

## Parts of Body

Some Reiki masters advise that seventh and third chakras should be avoided in Reiki healing, because these draw energy from the universe.If we put our hand there, energy will not enter and we will feel depressed. This not so, as per Paula Horan. These chakras require more energy because these supply to the other parts. Moreover these are blocked, third chakra by anger and seventh by worries because of its direct connection with the second. So Reiki must be drawn there. The author has also experienced that Reiki is essential for these chakras. If you feel depressed it means the negative energy of that chakra has come on the surface. Catch it and flick your hands and draw Reiki again. After a few days you will feel that depression has disappeared.

## Tree of Human Body

In Geeta and Upanishad human body is compared with a topsy - turvy tree. A tree has its roots in the earth and branches spread out in the atmosphere and grows by watering the roots. Roots of human - tree are in the head and its branches - limbs extend below. It will be nourished by drawing Reiki on 7th chakra and other head points.

6th chakra makes the cosmic aura, it is our spiritual body, the cause is the head and body is the effect. So treat the cause for general well - being. When a disease begins, it goes up within the body and when cured, it comes down and goes out of the body. It is advisable that while drawing Reiki we should begin from the crown chakra. Such is the method of taking the bath. At first wash your head and then come down slowly.

### Practical Aspects of Pranic Energy

Aura - touch–Every body receives and radiates pranic energy like breathing in the atmosphere but we are not conscious of these radiations. We can gain more with awareness.

Go towards a green and healthy tree. As you enter its shade. you will feel light, especially on the head. You have entered its aura and received the energy. By holding your hands with palms facing the sky, keep your fingers at distance of one inch from the trunk, stand for about half an hour. Watch the sensations in your fingers. You are receiving energy from its inner aura. Energy flows in and out through your finger tips. Tree also gains your energy. Now touch the trunk with palms. You will feel sensation in the palms. Embrace the trunk, you will feel light at the heart. Touch your fore head and you will feel light. Thank the tree, and come back slowly. Next day take a bucket of water and pour it around the trunk. Fold your hands and request the tree to give some energy if surplus . Be bare foot when under the tree. If you do it daily the tree will wait for you. Margosa tree (Neem) is the best for this purpose. If a T.B. patient stays all the day under it for one year he will be cured without any medicine. Fruit bearing trees are also good for this purpose. Avoid thorny tree like (acacia) Babul. It takes our energy and makes us weak. This is quite opposite to the margosa(neem) tree. Pine tree is also good.

Avoid Peepal and Banyan trees which give more energy than the man can withstand. You would observe that the round platform made of cement around the trunk of these trees get cracked because the roots emit too much energy.

Rose and Tulsi plants are useful in the surroundings of the house. Tulsi gives more energy and is anti - biotic. Rose plant emits balanced positive and negative energies.

**Aura - touch in human-beings**

Where ever we go we come in contact with human beings and can feel aura touch of each other. The same is the case when we are in the company of our own family members. We feel energetic in the company of the people we like. We lose energy when in the company of the persons whom we dislike.

If we cannot avoid the company of such persons, we should maintain good outworldly behavior. Keep in mind that every body is good and loving at the core of his heart and deserves respect, being a living wave of energy, but some people have rough behavior which is only outworldly. If any person reaches sixth chakra, he will become like Buddha. Pranic energy maintains our body in good condition but for permanent health and spiritual pursuit Reikei must be learnt and practised.

Universal energy moves like a wheel when it enters the chakras and goes out in the same way after use. Those circles of energy are received by others. Energy received by chakras is pranic, after Reiki initiation, Reiki is received by the seventh chakra along with pranic energy on the other parts.

Root chakra is nourished by taming non - vegetarian animals like dog and cat. Second chakra is nourished by taming vegetarian animals like cow, buffalo, goat, sheep, horse etc. Third chakra is nourished by the sounds of frogs. Fourth chakra by taming the birds like dove, parrot and peacock. Fifth chakra is nourished by the sounds of the birds.

The room or a place attains the personality of the persons who are present in it. If you go to a religious place your psychology will be different. Man is known by the company he keeps. We are attracted by the persons who have same vibrations. A child is attuned to the vibrations of his parents which may have been even two or three years prior to his birth. Once I had a chance to sleep in the room of a business man. In the dream I went to the bank to update the pass book. The clerk said he had no time to make so many entries and that I should make the entries myself. Through out the night I kept on making entries in the pass book. This had happened as the room was filled with the thoughts of accounts.

## Sea -Salt

Its use is essential in pranic healing but optional in Reiki. Sea salt absorbs negative energy, it is useful for L.B.P patients and harmful for H.B.P. Patients. Keep one liter of water mixed with a hand ful of salt in the room to remove the negative energy of the room. Keep your feet in hot water mixed with salt for 15 minutes daily for one month. You may take whole body bath with salt water and later with fresh water and continue for 4-5 days. You may also have whole body bath when depressed. You may continue taking bath at regular intervals and stop if you feel discomfort. Keeping the feet in the mud for 15 minutes daily is also useful and beneficial for inflamation or other problems. Contact with iron articles like chairs, buckets etc, takes away our negative energy. Reiki - cleansing is done by showering love and white light.

**Negative Energy** - Negative does not always mean bad. It is complementary and not opposite, as man is positive and woman is negative. Negative energy of diseases is grey and muddy in colour and creates flies, spiders, mosquitoes, bugs, germs, insects and bacteria. Positive energy if overdosed, becomes negative. Proceed from negative to positive and from positive to awareness.

## Positive Affirmation

People say "Think Positive". Is thinking in your control?. You may be successful for a few movements. Positive thinking will be imposed upon the negative. When the under-current is powerful it will throw away the positive. We live in the sphere of dualities, night is followed by day and vice versa. Positive and negative circumstances are a part of life. Life is incomplete with one. Positive circumstances give external power while negative ones give the internal.

Our life is planned by gods for us to balance and therefore, it is better to accept the divine order. An egoist will one day fall prey to inferiority complex. Don't think of good or bad deeds. Do your duty today. Self-respect is balancing.

Man has broken the cycle of dualities, invention of electricity has reduced night span. Indirectly humanity is suffering. Man has lost the sound sleep due to less darkness resulting in extreme anger and violence. Geeta chapter - II begins with accepting the dualities.

## Clapping

Clapping is common in religious devotional songs but had no logical and systematic base. Mr. Krishna Chand Bajaj (Madhuban, Pitampura, New Delhi) once heard in a sermon that clapping is good for health. He was about 80. He practised clapping sincerely but people ridiculed him. He did not bother. Some days later he felt he was cured of the diseases. He clapped one hour daily and introduced the same as the best exercise. Clapping activates the acu - pressure points of the hands.

**Method** - Sit on the chair or stand, feet touching the ground. Apply some oil to the palms and clap and then rest a while. Keep one hand fixed and clap with the other, if you are imbalanced. If left side is weak keep right hand fixed and vice-versa. Both hands represent the hemispheres of the brain. Left hemisphere of the brain controls the right side of the body and vice-versa.

Our different activities can be used as meditations and clapping is also part of it. During any activity our energy flows out and by sudden stop and it flows inward and we feel fresh. While clapping both palms should strike each other. Daily clapping for five minutes is sufficient along with other meditations.

Caution - Everything is not good for everybody. Clap slowly If you are a heart patient or suffering from H.B.P. All types of slow movements (slow dance) are good for the heart and H.B.P. patients and for the impatient persons.

Balancing by leg - stand or jump with one leg of the weak side of body.

## Mudras

This word is formed by two verbs mud and ramu which means enjoy and play and implied meaning is happiness. It also means to stop the energy of body by a special posture or by the fingers. Mudra is basically yoga of the hands. Four fingers and thumb represent five elements of our body, which supplement psychological and spiritual aspects. Diseases are cured by mudras.

**Thumb** - represents fire element and deals with- worry, purification, stimulatation and sixth chakra

**Index finger** - represents air element and deals with- grief, fourth chakra

**Middle finger** - represents space element and deals with- hastiness, fifth chakra

**Ring finger** - represents earth element and deals with- anger, first and third chakra

**Little finger**- represents water element and deals with- fear. Second chakra. Palmpit seventh chakra

Press thumb with other hand and pull apart. It avoids worry.

Press index finger with the other hand and pull apart, it avoids grief.

And so on... Right thumb represents sun and left Thumb moon. Joining thumb with the tip of any finger balances the element, Keeping thumb at the base of any finger, increases the element, Finger tip at base of the thumb, decreases the element in the body. With this theory you can make any required mudra. Stop mudra after the disease is cured. Certain mudras can be practised daily.

## Index Finger

This finger emits more energy, and is used in many ways. But it emits destructive energy and therefore, should not be used directly.

1. Some people put it on fore head in pranayam.
2. Some Reiki masters use it in drawing symbols in initiation, and clearing the space.
3. One of the Reiki Master advised to place this finger inside the ears for 10 minutes for instant freshness and energy.
4. Some people use for cleaning teeth. It does not show any harm since it is used for a short time. Harm is apparent if used for a long time.

**Self-experience**- About three years back my health required practising of Chandra Bhedi Pranayam (Cross Breathing First - Half)

Daily for 5 hours(one hour - five times) which I continued for two years. Normally this exercise is advised for five minutes only.

I used to close one nostril with the thumb and the other with the index finger. After a few days I felt itching in the nose which increased gradually. I also applied ointments with no result. some how I tolerated. But after two years I came to know that it was due to the touch of index finger.

**Experiment-** I conducted an experiment by plucking two fresh rose flowers. One flower was pointing towards my index finger and other away. After one hour I noticed that flower near my index finger faded whereas the one away was as fresh as before. I felt very sorry and guilty for hurting a flower as if I have hurt a child but my experiment proved that the touch of index is harmful.

Index finger is used as warning and for sudarshan chakra. It is a tradition that it should not be pointed towards young children and sprouting fruits.

Reiki symbols should be drawn by joining all the fingers. Index finger joined with others loses its bad effect, because thumb (fire) and the ring finger (earth) are purifying agents and the middle finger (space) weakens it by spreading its energy. Ring finger purifies. It is used in anointing the forehead and for blood test. Thumb or the middle finger can be used in place of index finger.

**Uses of Index Finger**

1. **Vayu Mudra** -Bend index finger and place it at the base of thumb keeping other fingers straight. It is good for gastric troubles.

2. **Apan Vayu Mudra** - Above mudra modified by touching middle and the ring finger with the thumb is called Apan Vayu Mudra. It cures the heart pain. Start with five minutes and increase gradually up to 40 minutes.

3. **Jnan or Dhyan Mudra** - Join the tip of index finger with the thumb for one hour. Thumb purifies its negative energy. It leads to knowledge, peace and meditation and can be practised daily.

4. **Anushasan (Discipline) Mudra** - Form both fists by bending all the fingers into the palms and placing thumbs on the ring fingers. Keep both fists on the chest for two minutes and feel the energy of all the 5 elements entering the chest. Keep eyes closed for two minutes. Open the eyes, remove fist slowly from the chest and stretch the index finger for two minutes. Close the index fingers and form the fists again and bring slowly close to the chest. This is one cycle. Repeat 6 times. Index finger expels negative energy.

**Other Mudras -**

5. **Apan Mudra -** (for removal of negative stuff from the body and mind). Join the middle and the ring finger tips with the thumb. By keeping index and little fingers straight the negativity is removed. Energy of fingers touching the thumb increases and returns to the chakras concerned and hits the brain chambers for enlightenment. Practise it for 40 minutes a day or 20 minutes twice.
6. **Balancing Mudra** - curve your fingers, clutch hands with each other, stretch both hands three or four times. Move elbows up and down.
7. **Veet Rag Mudra -** Sit on the floor or bed. Keep left hand on the lap and right hand over it for 40 minutes for circulatation and balancing of energy in the body.
8. **Ling Mudra -** Keep your right thumb straight to reduce fatness and to produce heat in the body, for solar energy, during cold weather. This is shivling mudra. You can keep left thumb up for lunar energy.
9. **Games** - volley ball. The use of left hand is less. It should be used more for balancing.

In mudras and yoga it is essential to join the universal energy for achievements.

## Sudarshan Chakra

It was a weapon and personal achievement of Lord Krishna - the warrior god. He used this weapon only once while killing Shishupal. It was not material at all. It was an energy circle looking like fire works. It is a subject for research. It was done by right hand stretched above the head, keeping three fingers closed in the palm and index finger stretched upwards, tip of the thumb touching its base. The author feels left hand should be stretched upward for receiving negative pranic energy where as in pictures left hand is shown downwards.

## More About The Chakras

**Root Chakra-** (Origin of the universe and the body). In Nasadiya Sukta - (Hymn of Cosmic Origin) of Rigveda it is said that there was pitch darkness in the beginning . It was all chaos and nothing was known. This darkness is mother energy, which creates universe, earth and our body. Einstein imagined about the dark energy which is yet to be experimented. It controls and creates the universe. The author thinks this as dark energy.

The original color of this chakra is dark black. By meditations of this chakra you see total or partial darkness like black animals and birds- buffalo, black cow, goat, crow etc. Seeing darkness is spiritually good as we witness the sleep. Black things are rarely seen in dreams. Sometimes you will see crowd, filth, animals like snake, dog, tiger, and dreadful events.

**Bi-location :-** This chakra is physically constructive as you can see your face or body in the dream or vision. When more powerful it can create two or more bodies. It happened with some persons when they were present in two places at the same time. They themselves were not aware of it. This can be done at will as an achievement. When Lord Ram Chandra returned to Ayodhya, all people of the city came to welcome him. He appeared in many forms and met every one at the same time. This was also the case with Lord Krishna.

**Awakening Kundalini -** Is a spiritual power (coiled energy - dormant, sleeping) in the vision of a snake. When awakened, one sees thousands of suns. Arjuna in Mahabharat saw such a lusture when Lord Krishana showed his universal personality and gave him divine insight (of sixth chakra).

One gains power along with happy family life. Its weakness causes the diseases of bones and formation of stone, constipation, loss of smell, memory and sleep.

**Root Chakra and Cycling -** when we ride a bicycle nerves of root chakra take the burden of all the body and are pressed. It is harmful especially for the young children.

This is a chakra of earth element and dominates the man who is interested in traveling around the world. If a man is religious he goes to pilgrimages, takes interest in building temples, monasteries, and idol worship.

It is directly connected with 6th chakra. Reiki given on it goes to 6th chakra and vice versa. If it is powerful, makes one fearless and enables him to create own kingdom or landed property.

**Root Chakra and Smell** - It is a chakra of the earth element, smell dominates it being the essence of the earth. In homoeopathy the smell matters in treatment. Vegetarian animals, men and gods like the smell of flowers, fruits, vegetables and sweets where as non - vegetarians animals, men and evil spirits, devils like the smell of meat, eggs, fish.

One who completely masters root chakra can produce any smell at his will. In the meditations of root chakra you will rarely experience smell.

Burning Loban or Gugal is useful for root chakra. Its smell is absorbed by this chakra and gives good health. Loban is used by Muslims and Gugal by Hindus during rituals.

First principle of Reiki - Honesty is associated with root chakra. Honest earning makes it strong. Dishonest and poor earnings make it weak.

**Root Chakra and Fear -** Seat of fear is root chakra. All chakras are extended up to the feet. Fear blocks the knee. Lack of love turns into fear. Fear is seen in the form of a snake and a lion. When we face the fear, root chakra becomes strong and if we do not, the energy block remains there. During meditation the author once saw an ugly toad - of muddy colour, emerging from the earth and was afraid and discontinued his meditation. The symbol of the snake is identified with kundalini. When all the energy channels are active the serpents seem to enter our body from all directions. This symbol increases fear and most of the meditaters stop their practice.

When we are afraid, our root chakra spreads a smell. Dogs and lions know our weakness, from the smell and attack us. Kundalini meditation of Osho eliminates fear.

Animals also know our fear by looking into our eyes. When 4th chakra, the seat of love, is fully developed, one becomes fearless like Lord Buddha and Lord Mahaveera and moves freely before these animals. As the fear shakes our body, so one can shake the earth, can bring an earthquake and vice-versa.

**Democracy and Fear -** Formerly people were terribly afraid of the kings and dictators. In democracy they are fearless, but some of them misuse freedom. However democracy is good for spiritual evolution.

## Root Chakra & Death

We live in the sphere of dualities. Here energy flows towards the opposite pole. Forces are in opposite pairs. Actually these are not opposite but are complementary to each other like day and night, man and woman, rest and work. Root chakra gives us birth and creates universe, after the full creation, energy moves towards opposite pole, the death, the dissolution of the world like the daily sleep. One who has enjoyed life does not fear death where as, the one who could not enjoy does not want to die and fears death. Ripeness is all. A fruit when ripe falls by itself as its grip becomes weak, a raw fruit can not be easily plucked. In western countries people enjoy life to full. They swim and go deep into the sea, fly in the air, jump from heights at the risk of their death.

Sigmond Frieud discovered that man has two emotions Eros and Thanatos. He desires to live long when happy, and to die when unhappy. Whenever we feel that life is worthless, our journey towards death begins. The people who are united with sixth chakra can leave body happily at their will.

A movement produces a sound. Every machine, when in operation, has its sound. A defective machine produces dull sound.

A good sound denotes health. There is a saying that sound mind has sound health.

Our body is full of musical sounds and so are the stars. Every chakra has its sound called seed mantra. It should be chanted for its awakening.

**Chakra Meditations - Root Chakra** - Its sound is lam, originally it was only la, M was added to move the energy upward. M is fixed in the sound of every chakra. The sound may be heard with a change. The author heard it as laos.

**Method :-**

1. Chant Lam orally, mentally and by the breathing. La and M two parts should be joined with each exhaling and inhaling.
2. Concentrate on the location of the chakra.
3. Draw Reiki at night as it is a seat of sleep.
4. Imagine its colour - black, bright dark (in books yellow or red is written - that is when its energy goes through ida or pingla)
5. Perrinial lock - shrink the nerves of root chakra and hold for a minute. Repeat it ten times, it melts the negative energy and releases it.

**Hara -** It is a chakra of relationship and enjoyments. Man is interested in developing relationships. Political leaders and religious masters are more interested in it. It blooms with moderate enjoyment but fades with lack of or excess enjoyment. Lack of enjoyments create worries and excess create greed. It is also a store of memories like root chakra. Water creates fluid in the body. Without fluid the body becomes weak and suffers from asthma, urinary disease, too much or no sweating. It is directly connected with the 7th chakra, covered with worries and greed .

You will see water, white objects, fishes, women, mirror, moon, cows in the dream. Its diet is vegetarian. It makes us fond of swimming and voyages. Its sound is vam. The author heard it as vach vach. Second principle of Reiki is concerned with "I will not worry today". Reiki given on it goes to 7th chakra and vice - versa. White things and atmosphere help it. One who fully activates this chakra, can produce water any where by collecting energy rays of water element. Or can bring sweating in the body even in winter.

**Sweating** - During the fever when the temperature comes down, the body sweats which means sweating is good for health. We can bear heat or cold if our body gives a normal sweat. If any part of body is devoid of sweating it is like a desert. There will be inflamation or other serious diseases of skin. One whose this chakra is weak he will have no or poor relations with women - including his wife, mother, sister, and daughter and the same applies for women.

**Navel Chakra -** It is red in color and by activation one sees the sun, fire, gems, popular persons. It is the seat of ego, anger and violence, and domination. If one is spiritual in nature then it gives a sense of abundance and leads to fourth chakra. It controls and gives energy to root and hara chakra as sun gives to the earth and moon.

For meditation chant its sound Ram. It is identified with the name of Lord Ram Chandra and his life which makes the chanting easy. The author heard aam aam and rom rom when its energy went to 5th and 6th chakra.Sound of Hoo Hoo is also useful. It goes down to the root and also serves the purpose of Uddyan Bandh (flying lock) exercise of the stomach. When anger is suppressed in the stomach, do it at once. It will release the negative energy of anger. Heat of suppressed anger causes swelling of intestine, liver and ulcers. It belongs to the third principle of Reiki - I will not be angry today.

By its power one can create fire. Quality of fire is appearance. By third chakra one can produce any appearance. Its sense organs are eyes, which inspire to read and write books, and motor organs are legs which inspires us in running and long walks.

**Anahat Chakra -** This chakra is sandwiched between the three chakras above and three below. It joins earthly and heavenly (Yin Yang) female and male energies and transform them. Here physical energy of root chakra becomes psychic energy of upper chakras and vice - versa. So it is a chakra of balancing, represented by six - pointed star formed by two triangles, one pointing above and the other below. This figure is useful in houses for absorbing positive energy and releasing negative.

It is a gateway of purity and emptiness. It is good when fully activated by meditations and love for humanity, otherwise the dominant negative energy of anger, violence, greed takes over and goes to the head making all aura muddy, creating diseases or destruction for others and makes a man devil. One sees angels and devils on this chakra.

This chakra takes a man "Far From The Maddening Crowd"(a novel written by Thomas Hardy). Here the man will either live alone or love only one friend. Lovers get sense of immortality and sacrifice their lives for each other.

It is green in colour and greenery appeals the man. He does not want to be aloof. This chakra inspires poetry, music and fine arts.Here the man is not a blind follower but decides himself on merits.

His decisions are emotional and not business - like. Here bondage surrenders, freedom begins, patience develops and the man becomes master of the situation as he does not want to dominate nor to be dominated. Its weakness causes dreams and power gives visions. Dreams are good if the chakra is least active.

Physical enjoyments are transformed into psychological ones like deeds in duty, joys and sorrows in serenity, anger, and sex into love, greed in satisfaction, ego in self respect, jealousy in service.

**Meditations** :- Its sound is Yam. The other meditations are games and other exercises with hands as in volley ball.

Raj yoga is free and creative. Raj yoga (Royal) begins with this chakra, and there is no need of technical yoga (Hatha yoga of postures). As love is taboo in society, it is linked with the devotion to God and inlcudes dancing, singing, clapping (kirtan). All types of human relations are imagined with the God - like father, mother, master, friend, foe, husband, wife and son which is nothing but ignorance and is a tradition in society. Poets wrote epics on these topics which are widely recited. Emotions remain suppressed.

A Tibetan saint Atisha has discovered a method which transforms sorrows into peace. We breathe in and out our aura thereby, the dust of our sorrows goes in and out every time. The negative energy can be turned into positive and is in line with positive affirmation because it is an effort, not a demand.

**Method -** Breathe in - see that your sorrows are transformed into peace and breathe out the same. With breathing you can add (Yam). After a few days your sorrows will disappear, and you can work for others. It is just like converting poison into medicine.Do it for 90 days.

Space of fifth chakra begins from here. There is a humming sound like that of bees - a space very small like the point of a needle (called Dahar in Upanishad) in the shape of a lotus flower. Search with-in and enter like an energy thread.

It belongs to the fourth principle of Reiki, I will love every body today.

It shows the images of flying birds, waving of flags and wind. When one masters it, he can create wind and vice - versa. When this chakra is fully activated in man's life, he joins the company of gods in the next birth and becomes capable of astral traveling.

Healing touch is extra-ordinary of a Reiki master who has reached in fourth chakra.

Love is momentary and limited to about five minutes during the whole life for those who have not reached fourth chakra.

**Fifth Chakra -** Throat is the main joint and all others are linked with it. It avoids congestion and keeps them healthy. In fourth chakra our energy is turned into permanent love. In fifth chakra, the seat of wisdom, one is filled with the permanent desire for self realization. Sorrows and tension turn into non-attachment. It is a chakra of purification, creates elixir of life called Somarasa in Veda, Homa in Persian and Abe Hayat or Abe Jam Jam in Urdu. A liquid from Bindu chakra (7th chakra) drops in it and is divided into poison and nectar. If the chakra is active it retains the nectar and expels the poison and man remains healthy and young in old age also. Certain persons digested poison as per history. Sipping and sucking is meditation of seventh chakra for this purpose.

A child takes milk from its mother's breast, which nourishes the body and makes internal brain active. The children who are deprived of their mother's milk and fed by spoon remain poor in physical and mental health. In Vedic rituals a spoonful of water put on the palm is sipped for 3 times saying that it is nectar which is only symbolic.

Osho has said, if you play act of sucking for 40 minutes daily you will someday realise the elixir of life dropping from your head into the throat. St. Kabir has said "O! Saint stay in sphere of sky (inner head) there nectar drops, there is always happiness, drink the nectar". In urdu literature it is called wine (inner) but people take it for outer one.

Ham is sound for chanting. Ha sound will also do. Hari, har are other sounds. Laughter, using the word ha, spreads energy in all joints and removes joint pain, creates happiness, is easy and also good for health. It is an exercise of the stomach and saves from many diseases including that of heart. This is the chakra of speech, expression and communication. It belongs to the fifth principle of Reikei, "I will be grateful to every body today". By its mastery we can send and receive thoughts from a distant place. One sees meditators on this chakra.

**Sixth Chakra -** This chakra is called Mahakasha. It has greater space (energy) as compared to that of 5th chakra. One gets enlightened and sees enlightened persons on this chakra.

Its sound is Om, heard as Amen by Christian and Muslim mystics. All balancing exercises are its meditations. Draw Reiki and chant Om. Energy enters from back of the head, vibrates in the front and there after with long practice in the whole body. Its color is indigo. Meditate in the open by lying down and looking at the clear sky either in the early morning or in the evening for one hour. Constant looking for one hour at the mirror, darkness, lamp, natural scene, a tree, a wall or a roof are its other forms of meditations. It belongs to 6th principle of Reikei "I will balance my life today".

**Seventh Chakra -** It is called Chidakash - conscious space. Its color is violet and meditation is humming - a subtle form of Om. Practise humming at least for 30 minutes (See Osho's Nad Brahma meditation).

This chakra is called Bindu - means drop. Bind - means to divide. Here universal consciousness is divided into personal one. In root chakra kundilini is solar (thousands of suns). In this chakra kundilini is lunar - thousands of moons. Here different types of lightenings are seen. The books recommend chanting of the sound mantra for five minutes for each chakra but it can be done as much as one can do. Meditate on each chakra for one month. Reflexology deals with the chakras of the foot sole. Its method is massage.

The fishes which are born at bottom of the sea can not come to the surface as their body is accustomed to bear the weight of water above their body. The body of such fishes burst when they come to the surface. The fishes which are born on the surface can jump to sea shore. One has to judge him self and proceed with dominating chakra. The frequency of these chakras increases as we proceed to upper chakra.

## Imagination of the colors in chakras

In some books, during practicing of yoga, one is told to imagine the color of the chakra. Imagination is not helpful in the beginning. You should practise the meditations of the chakras - chant their sounds (mantra) draw Reiki upon them, you will see their colors yourself and realise that imagination was not required. Then you will remember the colors. Imagination will be poor, impotent and misguiding with less practice, thereby, inviting fear of fault.

Once the author was attending a yoga camp and the teacher was addressing about the imagination of blue color for peace and calmness. The persons attending the class practised it for half an hour. One lady could see white color instead of blue in spite of her strong determination. She informed the same to the yoga teacher. Yoga Teacher said even white colour was good which was a poor consolation.

Whenever you begin a meditation, you will see the symptoms of a particular chakra which is dominant in you. Leave that chakra and go to another chakra either above or below. Most of the yoga teachers learn yoga by going through the books and teach yoga with little or no experience.

**Yoga - Postures -** These are related to chakras but people practise like random exercises. Even exercises are spiritual if done in an order from top to toe as proposed by master Choa Kok Sui. Every chakra has its gland, organ and a part of body. Exercise of that part is a yoga posture. For information see yoga books. (Chakra healing by Lis Sympson - London )

### Spiritual Exercises are Substitute of Yoga

Invoke God else it may be dangerous - If God is not invoked evil spirits will enter the body. These exercises pave the way for energy from head to the feet.

1. Exercise of the head - stand up move your eyes ten times in clockwise and then 10 times anti clock wise.

2. Neck - move neck forward and backward ten times each, and then side ways and around also ten times each.
3. Put your hands on the shoulders - rotate your elbows ten times clockwise and 10 times anti clockwise.
4. Hips - move hips ten times in each direction, clock wise and anti clockwise.
5. Jogging - 5 minutes.

For further details go through "Miracles of Pranic Healing" by master Choa Kok Sui.

Exercise of joints - move around wrists and legs. Shrink all parts of body and let the same loose.

## Enlightenment & Brain Chambers

According to yoga there are six chambers in the brain connected with the six chakras. First and second chakras are connected with the chambers of the back brain, third in the middle head, sixth further to it, fifth and fourth in front head. Energy of chakras activated by meditations and Reiki goes up to the brain chambers and is received if open, otherwise returned with a jerk, to the chakras. The chambers can be opened by repeated knocks of chakra energy from below and by Reiki from above. Mudras are also helpful. Energy of five elements is checked in mudras which flows to the chakras and chakras in turn send it to the chambers. Mudras and Reiki activate the hemispheres and balance yin yang energies. When you feel the chambers are being activated - sheershasan - a posture in yoga (standing on the head) is useful for two minutes, otherwise it is harmful. Pressure of blood breaks the small tissues and makes our mind dull. In yoga people do it daily without knowing this fact. Sheershasan is called the king of the postures but do it only when needed. When all these chambers are opened, lighted and full of energy the man is enlightened and becomes Buddha.

## Balancing Energies

Nature has provided all human beings with facilities for balancing but culture and society has caused hindrances. Balance of breath is disturbed by tension, which ultimately affects the body. Close the nostril which flows more with a piece of cloth. Achieving and maintaining balance is an important aspect in life.

### Balance of breath

We breathe by one nostril at a time. Breathing by both nostrils causes ill health. A healthy and cheerful man breathes for 90 minutes alternatively by each nostril. Imbalance creates tension, action and rest of poor quality and therefore, we should balance the breath.

Second step - we should be able to hold breath in and out for equal time. Generally people hold more within and less out. Breath should be deep all the day. Balancing is as difficult as weighing live frogs, two or three frogs always keep on jumping. Enjoy it as a play else you will lose the game, because universal energy is playful. The nature helps if you are sincere.

The balance when achieved and maintained for a few years reveals the secrets of life and universe.Balance of five elements of food, in three humors–phlegm, air, black and yellow bile, and in activities is also required. Now a days a person who tops in health, wealth, studies, sports and other activities is respected most. Balancing is must. Reiki also does the same purpose. It is the final achievement and the transcendence of dualities.

### Meditations of Balancing (of Sixth Chakra)

## Constant Looking on the Nose Tip

1. Do it without mirror and with eyes half closed. Remove spectacles if you are wearing. It seems simple but actually is difficult. When we look at the nose tip we see only one side of the nose either right or left. This is not our aim. You may be successful for a few seconds and then you will not see the nose because you have reached the inner soul. When balance is achieved, duality

ends, and awareness is attained. When there is balance of Ida and Pingla channels at the root chakra you will feel light because third force sushumana begins to work. Here we reach above the duality.

While standing or walking your body is imbalanced, weight of the body is more on one leg and shoe sole of that side gets pressed and wears more. You always hear from one ear. If you try to balance, the energy will go to the other ear and there will be same imbalance. When balanced you will feel that there is no need of ears to hear. Similarly when there is a balance in standing you will feel that there is no need of ground or feet to stand on.

When you walk you do not look straight but look either right or left. Look straight for balance. Our weak side of body suffers from diseases. About 80% of people are imbalanced and need exercises of one side only either right or left.

In china much work is done in discovering the methods of balancing. For example do this exercise with a partner. Press palms of both the hands against that of your partner. There should be cooperation and not the competition. The idea is not to win or lose. If you are more powerful you should give chance to your partner to press more and vice - versa. Stop when you feel balanced.

2. Face palms of your hands upwards and let your partner put his hands facing downwards above yours. You should push upwards and he should press down. Stop when the balance is reached and vice versa.

**Whirling and spinning**- If left side of your body is weak, move around yourself clockwise, to activate your right hemisphere. It is called spinning. If right side of your body is weak, move around yourself anticlockwise to activate your left hemisphere. It is called whirling. Stop immediately when you feel giddy. Whirling is positive charge and spinning is negative charge. Balance yourself according to your need. The balance leads to enlightenment.

Jalaluddin Roomi was enlightened at the age of eighteen by whirling. He used to do it as a play from the very childhood. He is founder of whirling amongst the Sufies. In south India people spin around themselves four times as a religious activity.

Balance yourself by walking straight, right or left according to your need. If your left side is weak walk towards to the right side and turn around yourself and walk towards the same side and vice - versa.

## Emptiness

"Blessed are those who are poor in spirit" **- Bible**

St. Kabir says "My mind enjoys poverty". Here poverty means emptiness. People take its literal meaning. There is almost nothing in the house of a poor man where as the rich man has every thing what ever he wants. People think that God loves poor people more than the rich as they are closer to the God which is not true. Basic needs of a man should be fulfilled by him with his normal efforts and with self- respect. If a poor man is worried about his needs, loses self respect at every step, he can never be satisfied and will be away from God. God helps those who help themselves.

Fulfilment cannot exist without emptiness but emptiness can exist without fulfilment. You build a house to live, but a house can exist without you.

Saint is called a faquir in Urdu language which means a person who has entered emptiness. These days he is called a beggar.

In Upanishads sentences such as " I am Brahman", " I am That", "You are That", "This soul is Brahman". "All is Brahma" were uttered by those who were in ecstasy of vastness and, eternity.

## White Light Imagination

" I know the purush of white colour, beyond darkness. One who knows it transcends the death. That is the only way to salvation." **- Veda**

Common man imagines different colours as in the case of chakras. If you are a Reiki channel and second degree holder you must have seen white light with a little blue tinge. It is taught in third degree but you can practise even earlier. White light is generally seen as it is also the color of second chakra. If you cannot see the light immediately, you will feel at least the Reiki entering your seventh chakra which will serve the purpose.

**Method** - Sit or lie down silently in a closed room, switch off your mobile phone. Invoke Reiki and imagine its white color above your head, if necessary touch your 7th chakra and draw Reiki. Then begin, and feel the energy entering and filling every part of your body, from head to toe. Do it slowly and patiently. Master Choa Kok Sui describes it as Twin Heart Meditation. Begin from 4th Chakra and then with 7th. For details see his book "Miracles of Pranic Healing". White light takes down our negative energy to the earth and fills us with fresh energy. White is the dress of gods. If you wear white dress and fill the room with white light it will be beneficial. White light can be had by a torch on the chakras and whole body for cleansing.

There is a person in Malad (Bombay) who claims to cure all diseases. When he treats the patients, he throws white light on the Chakras in the front part of body with an instrument of light. He points the light at the diseased part of body and passes energy waves by his hands with scattered fingers moving up and down like aura sweeping. He has learnt this art from the Literature of Lord Mahaveera, the founder of Jainism.

Sky is full of energy. Imagine to place yourself in the sky for half an hour and you will feel energetic. Energy flows from the root chakra and goes to seventh chakra.

**Dragon Breath - (Kapal Bhati - the Glow of the Fore Head):-** It is a means to balance breath in and out. Most people do it wrongly. Breath should be thrown out fast and repeatedly for 10 minutes. People take in fast breath. Due to our accumulative nature, we breathe in more and hold for a longer period than to breathe out and hold. It is the case with 70% people. This is useful for them but not for every body. When we stop the energy produced by quick breathing, it hits the heart and makes it weak because our 4th Chakra is blocked with grief and its thoughts. To avoid it, laugh immediately for 10 minutes, laughter may be artificial. It will pave the way for energy to go up to the throat and there by saves the heart. Then stop. Meditation begins. Sustain it as long as you can.

Indian classical songs and games like Kabaddy are the substitutes of dragon breath.

## Controlling The Mind

Conscious mind is just like an executive work in - charge. It comes to existence when we begin any work and it ends with the work. So there is no question of controlling it. Necessity of controlling is only of the subconscious mind. Controlling means supressing the thoughts and emotions which seem powerful. Controlling the mind is a very popular saying in our country. Man can control it only when he is strong. When he becomes weak, emotions like anger burst out. Normal catharsis of emotions is obtained by reading literature or seeing pictures and films. This control goes on for lives together. Controlling hinders the spiritual growth. Sixth Chakra is the Master of the mind (mind generally means sub conscious mind.). So long as we are below 6th Chakra the energy waves of mind go on, we are used by them just as a weak master by adamant servents. When we reach Sixth Chakra we can use the mind as an instrument to live worldly life or dissolve it for further journey.

## Desires

We have noted that desire is the major energy block. One desire, fulfilled or not, gives birth to another desire. Life always seems incomplete and the desire to complete it leads to the cycles of rebirth. You can understand it by the example of daily life. At the time of sleeping, you think over the actions and achievements of all the day. If something remained undone or half done, you say I will do it tomorrow. When you wake up, you start with the same unfulfilled idea. This process goes on till death. Cycles of birth are as the cycles of days in present life. When there is a repetition it is almost impossible to come out. This type of journey is almost eternal. One has to jump to the upper chakra. At the age of 22 I went to my village to meet my uncle. Aunt was sitting with a child in her lap. It was her son.

After thirty years I again went there. I have undergone many changes. But she was still sitting with a child in her lap. I was wonderstruck. Now it was her grandson. So people do not know about any progress. Generally people live in first two Chakras. As fish jumps out of the sea so man jumps out of the earth and goes to the moon. It is the same thing. When we reach fifth chakra (the chakra of wisdom or viveka) we are filled with the intense desire for self realisation and after much struggle and trouble we enter emptiness. This is the last desire.

## Company of Angels

### "May We Enjoy the Company of Angels" - Veda

Man is a link between the animals and gods in the evolutionary process. As man has broken connections with the animals so has he done with the gods. Man has come from the animal life and his destiny is god and further to be a Buddha. There are such currents of energy in his chakras.

Vedic rituals and prayers are all for calling the gods. Call compels an answer. Gods do come and exchange energies with human beings, as we do with the animals. It is not difficult to call gods. After second degree Reiki you draw the distant symbol along with others, give Reiki for three months, the god will some day come to you. For this purpose you should know the name of god. Ancient gods have left their bodies and entered once in human body and attained moksha by meditations.

Such gods will never come back. Some other gods may come, seeing your sincerity. Man is accompanied by gods and devils. If he is cent percent honest, gods accept him and devils leave him for ever, and vice-versa. In Reiki practice and initiations, Gods, spiritual guides and ascended masters take part. They correct our mistakes, and guide through images. Invoke those gods and you will feel their presence someday. They come at once by astral travelling.

There are hidden forces behind life. When we take meals gods or devils are present. Smell of the food is sufficient for them. The gods are present between 10 AM to 11 AM. and 6 PM to 7 PM. and the devils between 1 PM to 3 PM. and 10 PM to 12 midnight. In India gods have abandoned us since we take our food at the time of devils.

Qualities of gods are like those of human beings. Some are warriors, some are engineers, some are doctors etc. In Faith - Healing the healer invokes God and requests Him to send a healing angel for the patient. The angel comes and stays with the patient until he recovers his health. If a patient is near to death, the angel will not come. Devils are opposite of gods, they are full of negative energies for enjoyments at any cost. They are cruel, selfish, and violent, and ugly. Their aura is muddy. They have no halo. At the end they surrender to the enlightened persons and enter divinity.

## Evolution

The Love energy of Reiki is the base of the creation and the same is the cause of dissolution also. Loving energy goes to the matter and comes back to itself. This is the eternal play of hide and seek, a Leela, a mono drama. Coming down to the matter is descending order of energy. It is devolution, it is Reiki. When energy comes back to itself is evolution. It is called Kundalini in yoga, the ascending order of energy. Both currents of energy are to be used. Now a days we are in the ascending order. The process of evolution is as follows.

Rock-Moss-Plants-Insects-Animals-Human beings-Gods-The Buddhas. When animals show human qualities, they enter human life. Man may be from a frog, cow, horse, elephant, parrot, crow, etc. Face of men resemble those of animals and reminds them of their past life.

Chetak - The horse of Maha Rana Pratap is famous for its faithfulness and patience in Indian history. In the war with Mogals, the horse was wounded badly. Maharana lost the war, and he fled away on his horse.

There was quite a wide stream on the way. Two Mogal soldiers chased him. The horse jumped and crossed the stream, and fell dead. The soldiers came but their horses could not jump over the stream. Horse Chetak was wounded, lame and fatigued but was active till death. This horse had the human quality and such horses are born as men.

## Dark Energy Imagination

At the time of sleeping imagine that darkness is rising like clouds from the root chakra of your foot - soles and gradually coming to your root chakra of the body through both legs. And from that chakra rising towards the head filling all the body. It will arouse fear sometimes in the form of some wild animal. Face it, that animal is yourself of the past life which gives good health.

## Healing

Literally, healing means to cure, but healing also means to give energy to proceed further. A healthy, medically fit and mentally sound man will say, "I need no healing, I am not sick, I need not learn Reiki." He is wrong. A healthy man will grow spiritually very fast. Every body needs Reiki, even the gods. So long as one is not enlightened he needs Reiki.

King Yudhishtra wanted to enter heaven with his dog. The dog was not allowed. Yudhishtra was determined to go with it or not to go at all. A healing angel came, healed the dog, brought it into human form and then into a spiritual being. Thus dog was able to go to heaven with him. This story may be symbolical but it denotes the power of healing. It is very slow in gradual process, we can speed it up.

Now a days, capable Reiki masters are healing the earth. The calamities are reduced to ten percent only as against the forecasts. We hope that the earth will be saved from destruction.

## Reiki Master

A Reiki master must be healthy, cheerful, respected, educated, having a happy family life. He must have at least five years practice of Reiki. After three years practice of second degree initiation, he is able to draw abundant energy from the universe. In three years, symbols are drawn on the chakras for more than one thousand times. Then he can enjoy the sense of abundance and can claim to cure diseases. There was a custom in China that a capable doctor cures only by his energy, he does not give any medicine.

## SUBCONSCIOUS MIND

The subconscious mind is a group of our unfulfilled desires, it is our past and in imagination we project it in the form of a modified future. We miss the present moment. All energy, knowledge, beauty and truth is in the present moment.

**"May God give me supreme knowledge today".**

**"May God give me supreme energy today"**

**"May God give me happiness today"**

**- Veda**

Essence of today is present moment. Peak experience of life is in the present. Thoughts belong to the past and future. Present is the only reality. Quality of present moment is "I am". In all changing activities of life concentrate upon "I am", chant it. Do not think further. This experience is eternal. When we are conscious of our doings, and aware of your being, there is a deep peace in it. Every today contributes to our final achievement.

**Thus yesterday, today, tomorrow come**
**They hustle one another and they pass.**
**All our hustling morrows only make**
**The smooth Today of God.**

**- Theocritus**

## Reiki Mother : The Vastness

From the very childhood
In your love was wrapped,
In the desert or the wood
Happily I clapped.

I saw you all around
Standing on the hills.
Lying on the ground saw
In the sky with the thrills.

At the sleeping time.
Vastness of the dark;
If you are aware.
You can easily mark.

Alone, alone, all alone.
If you are not bore
Vastness is shown
On the sea - shore.

On the journey people go
In the east and west
With every body Sun doth glow
Always at the rest.

So long as we need to hear
To speak or to see.
We are far far away
From the sea of energy.

1

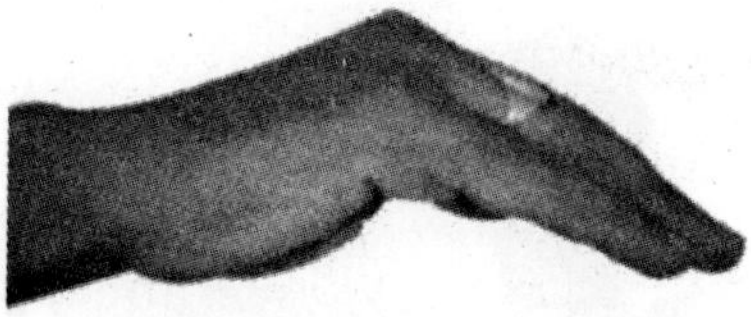

Spoon Shape Hand

2

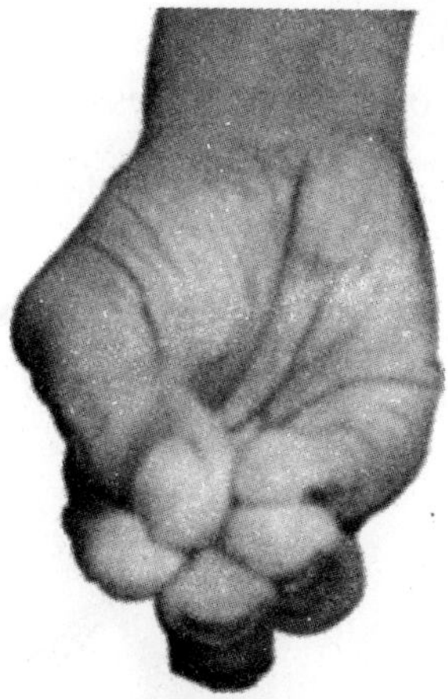

Curled fingers

# PARTS OF BODY

3

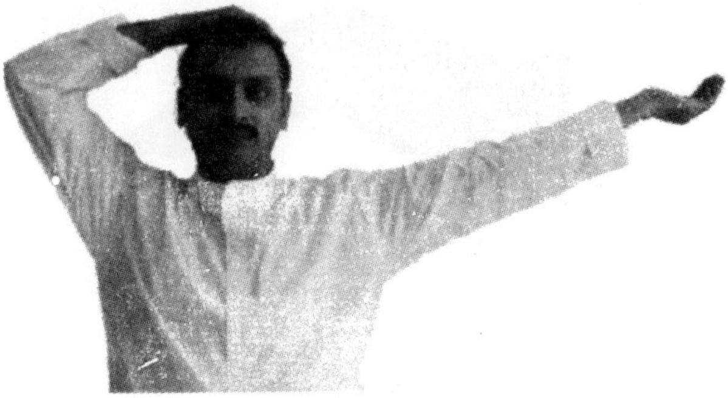

Reiki on Crown - (Bless yourself)

4

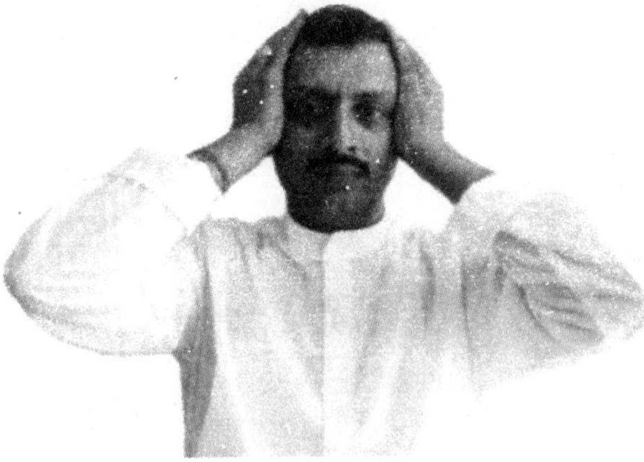

Temples

5

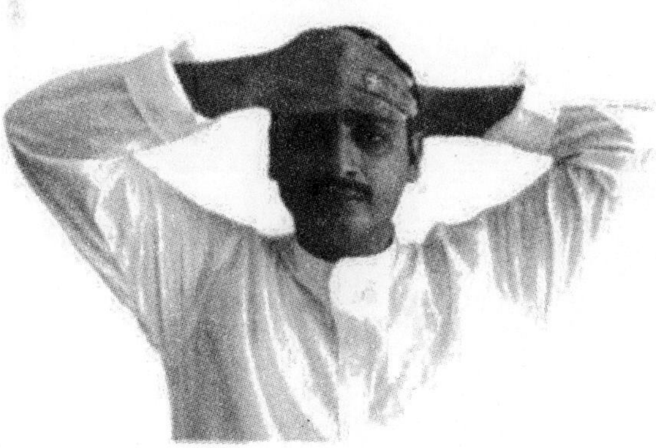

Sixth Chakra - Front and Back

6

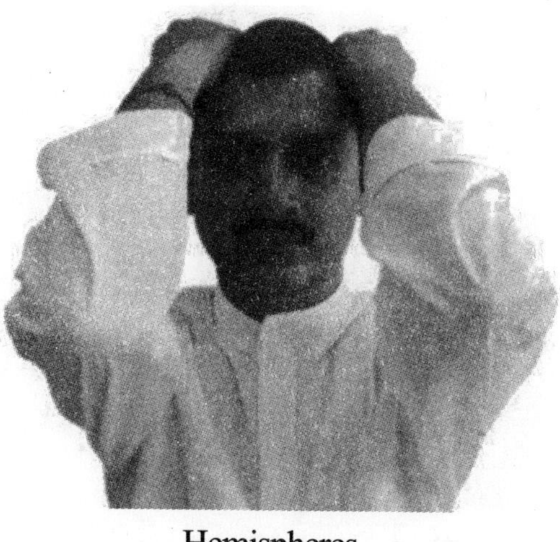

Hemispheres

7

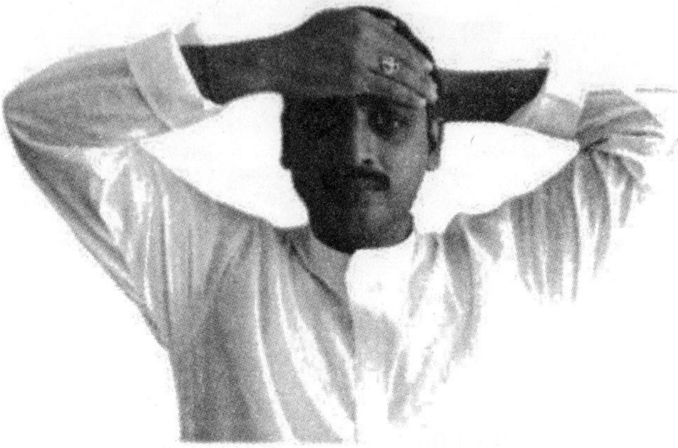

Brain Chambers

8

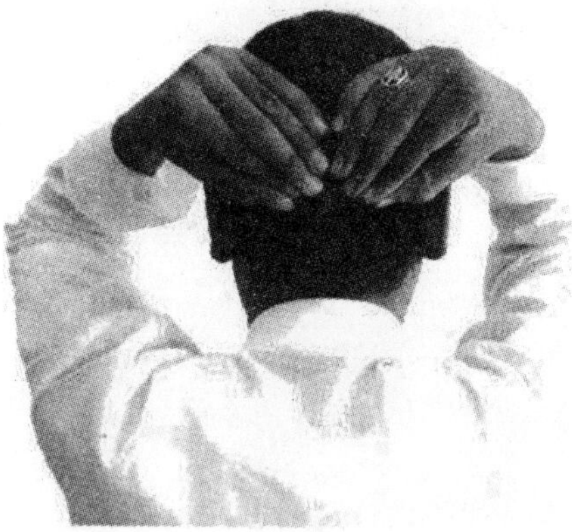

Back Head- Chambers

9

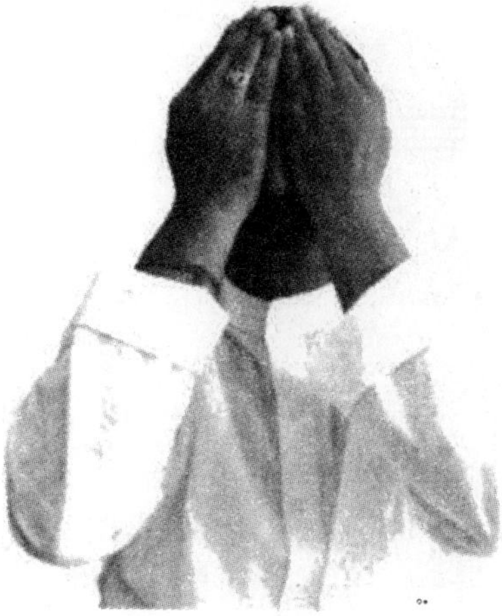

Eyes

10

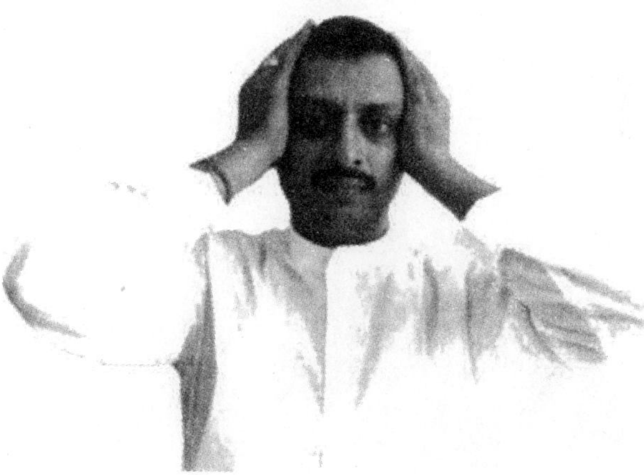

Ears

11

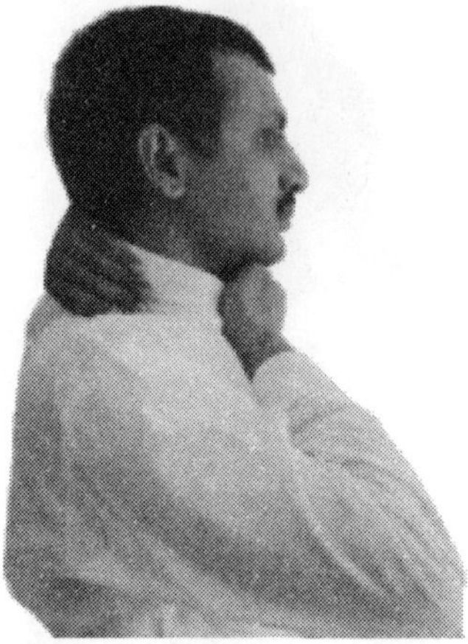

Throat Front and Back

12

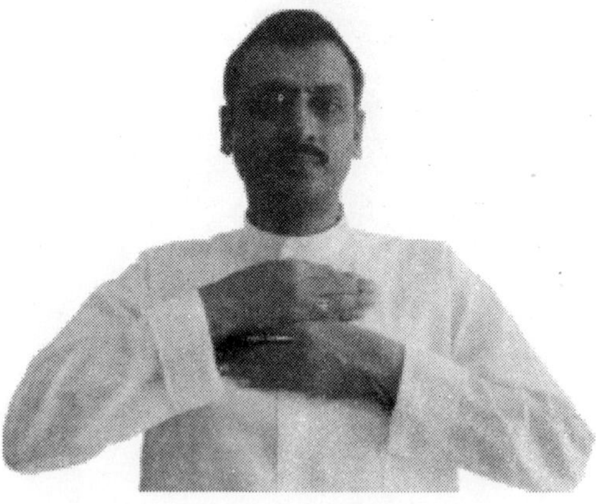

Thymus and Fourth Chakra

13

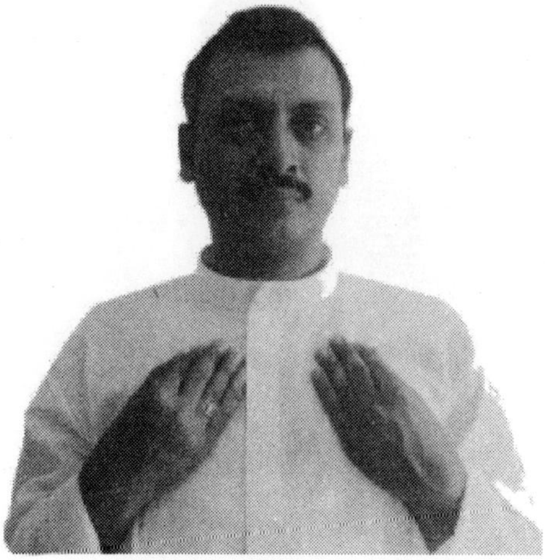

Lungs

14

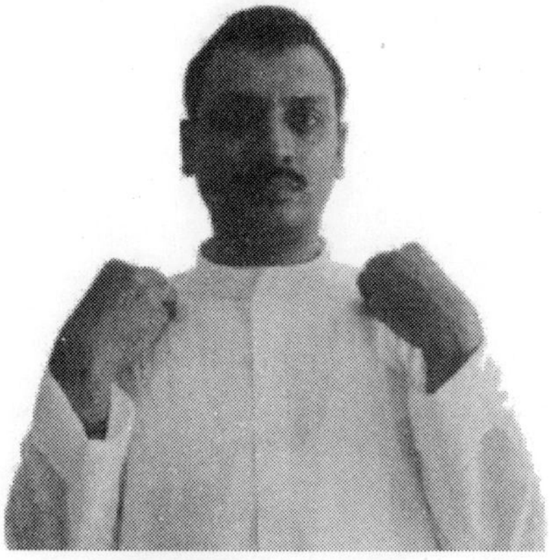

Shoulders - Curled Fingers for Pointed Parts

15

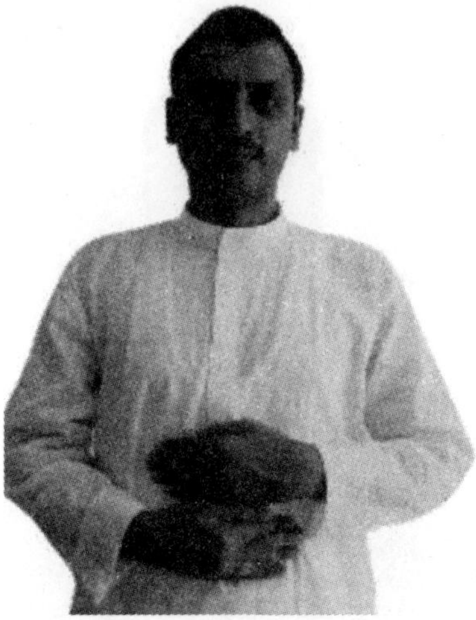

Navel and Pancreas

16

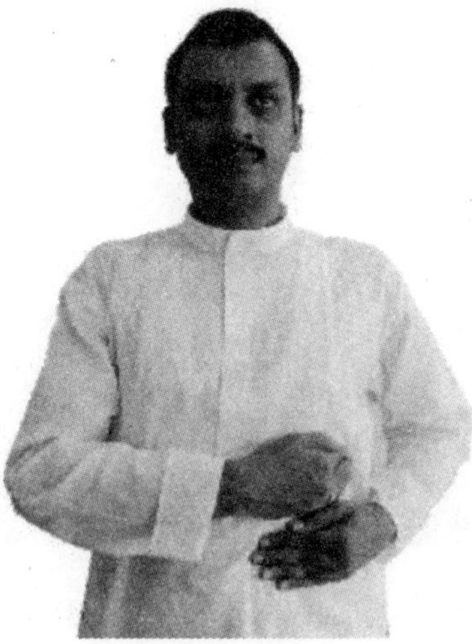

Spleen

17

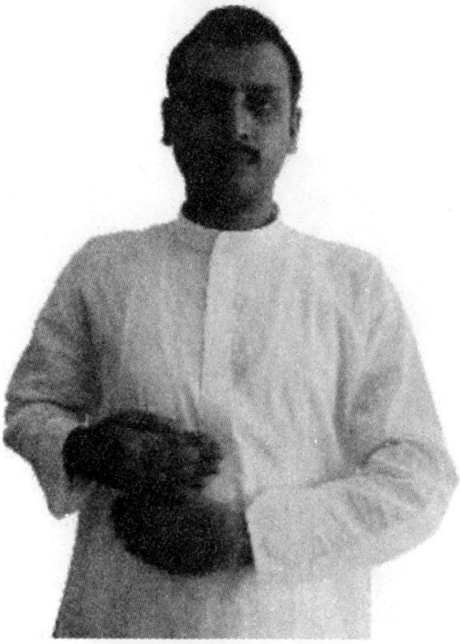

Liver

18

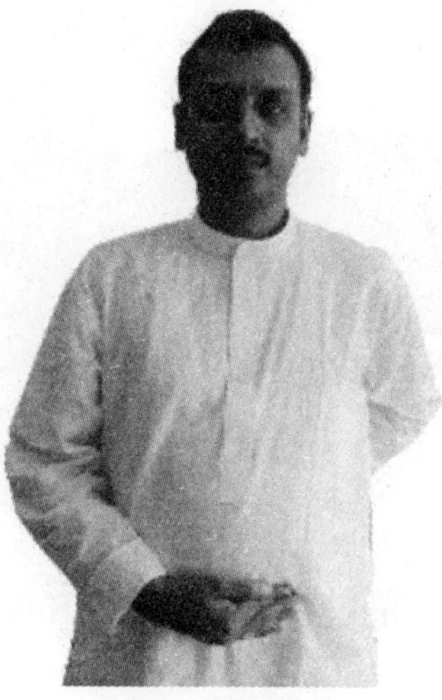

Hara Front and Back

19

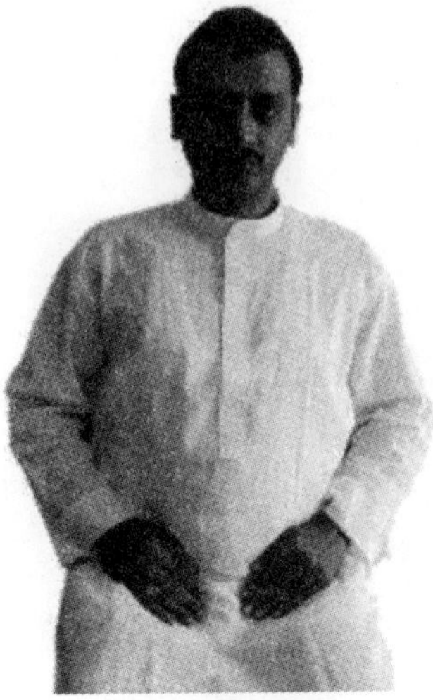

Thigh Joints

20

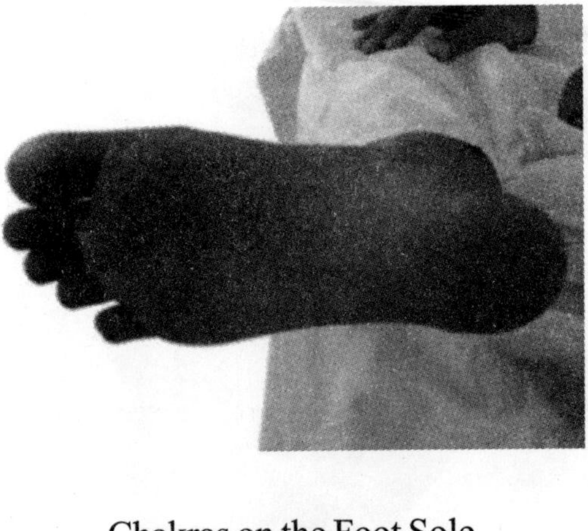

Chakras on the Foot Sole

21

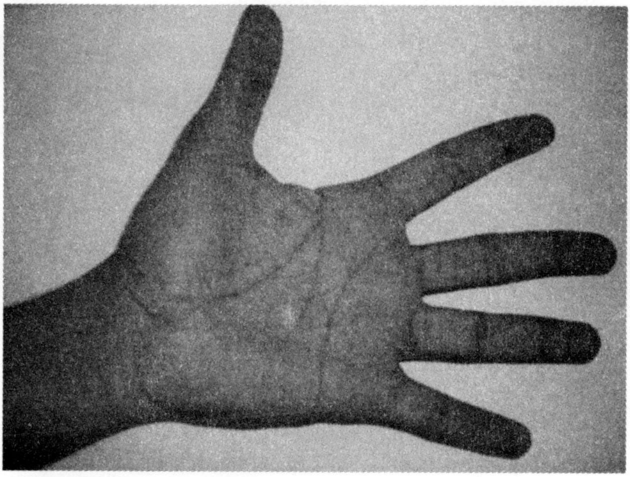

Chakras in the Hand

22

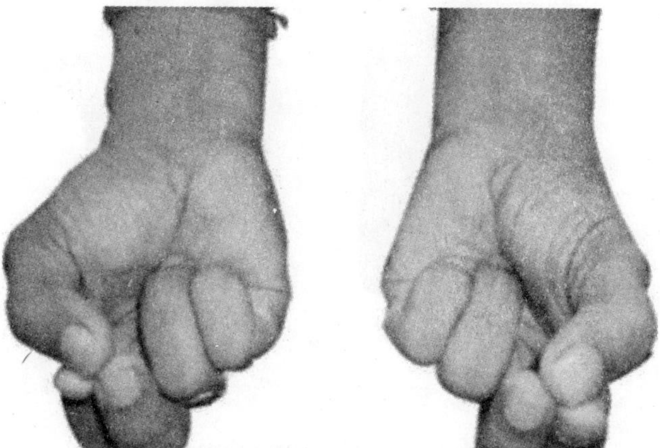

Kuber Mudra - for abundance

23

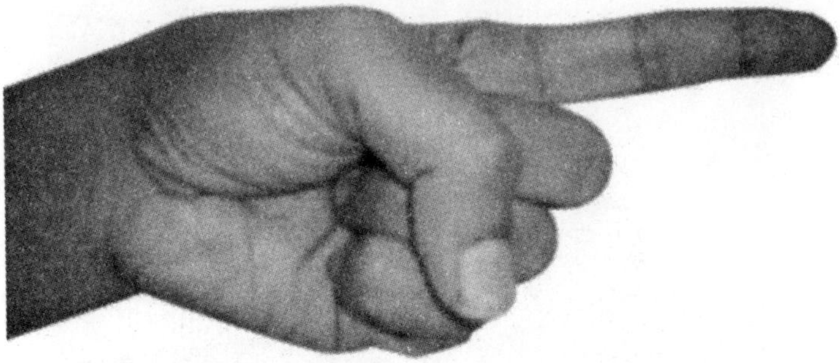

Index Finger

24

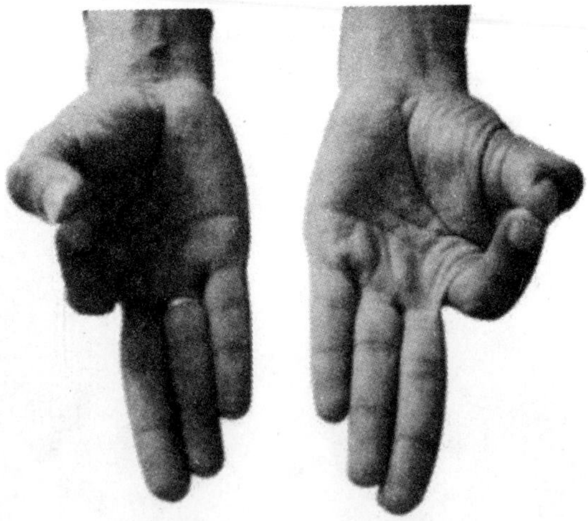

Jnan Mudra- for Knowledge and peace

25

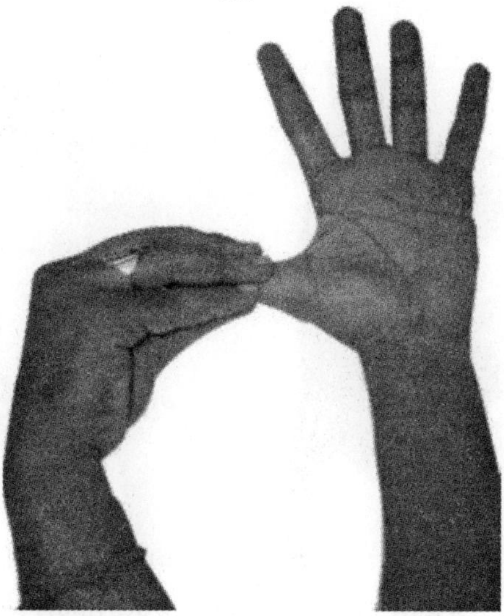

Arun Mudra

26

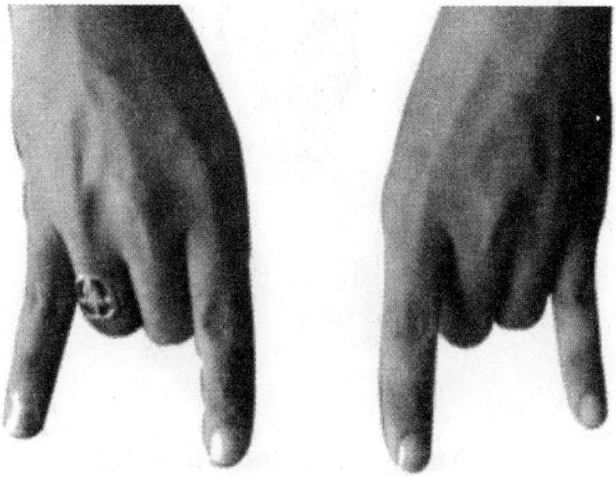

Apan Mudra

27

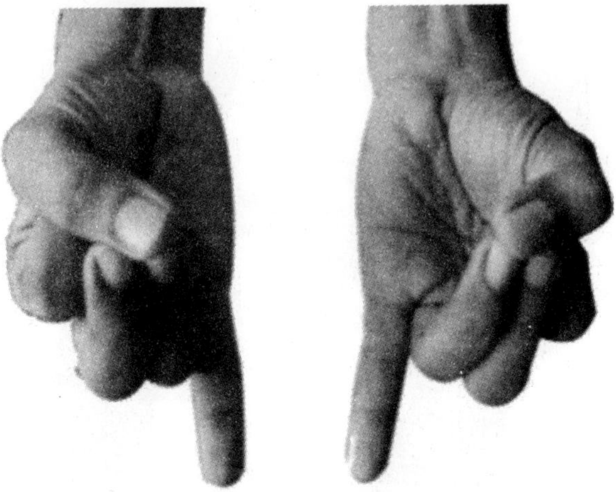

Apan Vayu Mudra - stops heart pain

28

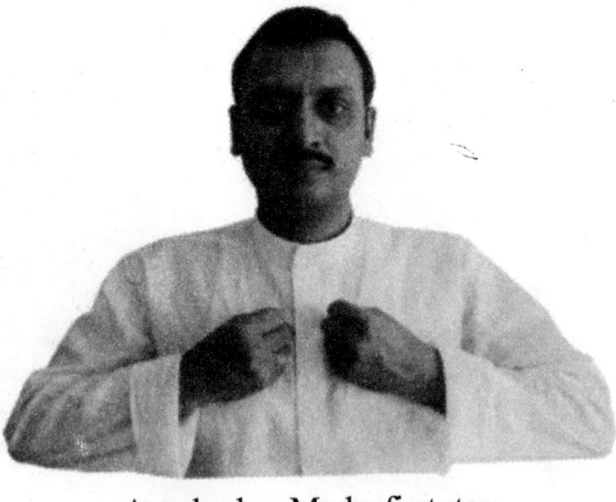

Anushashan Mudra first step

29

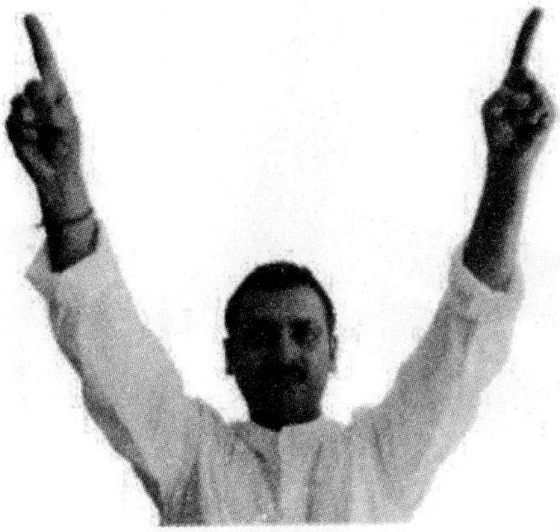

Anushashan Mudra Second Step

30

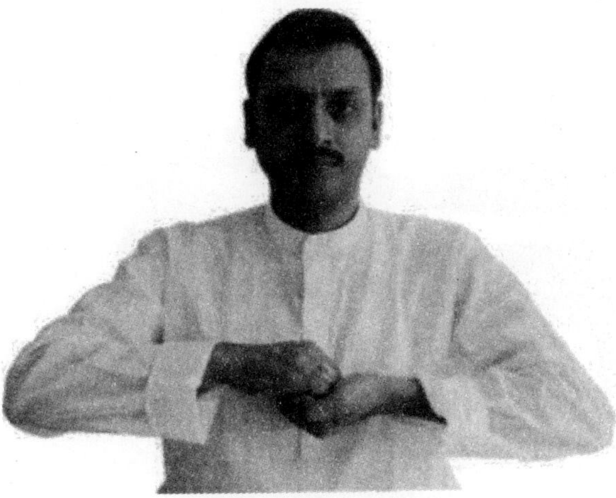

Balancing Mudra

31

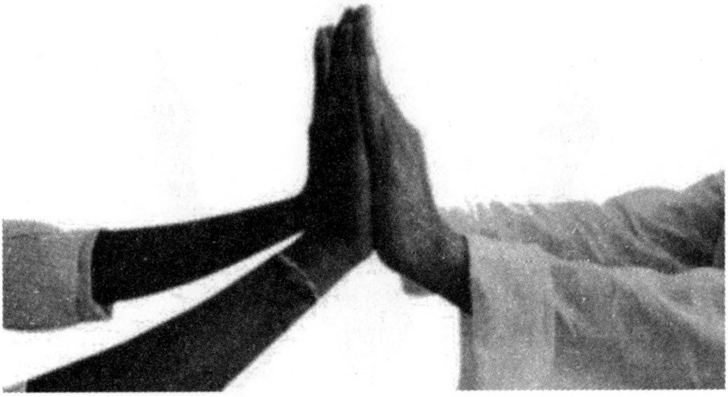

Balancing Energies - 1

32

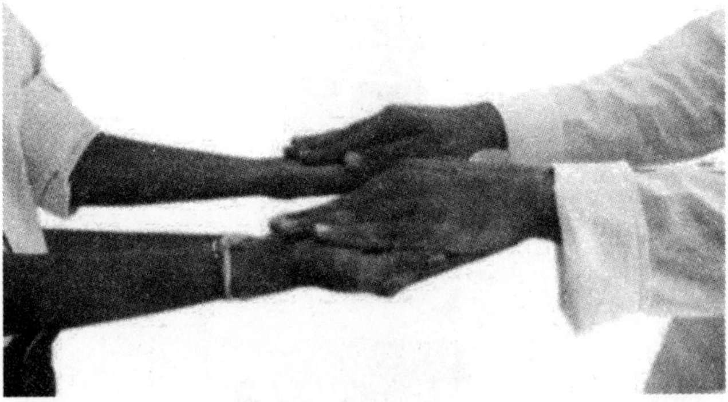

Balancing Energies - 2

33

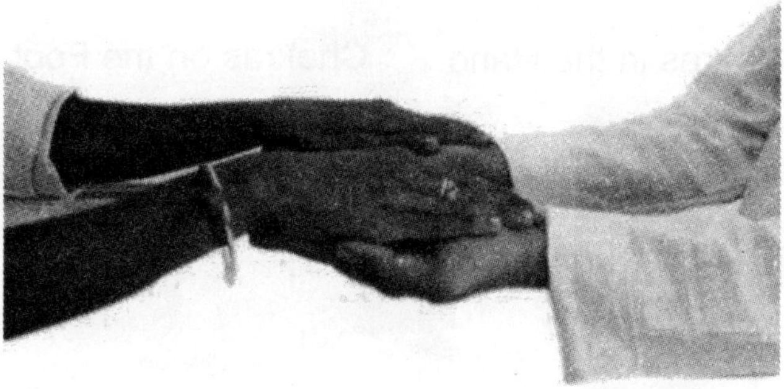

Balancing Energies - 3

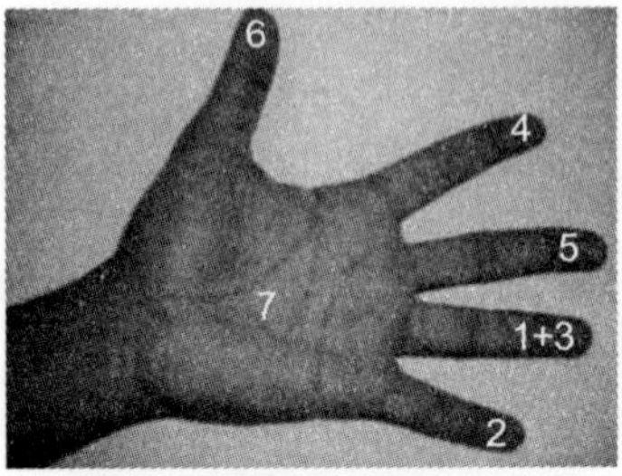


Chakras in the Hand

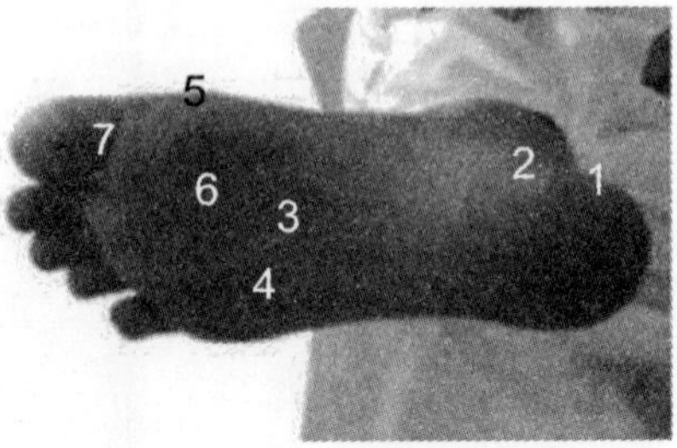


Chakras on the Foot Sole

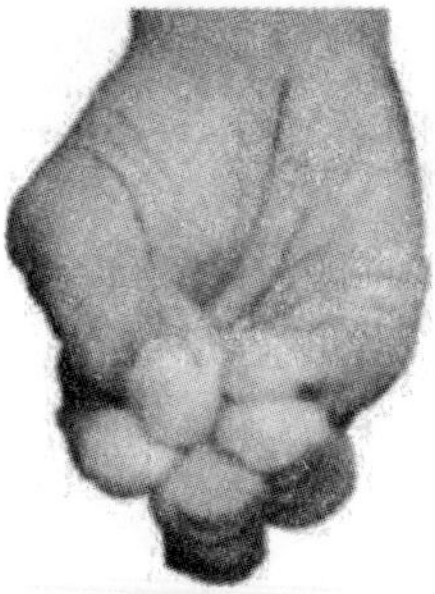

Curled fingers

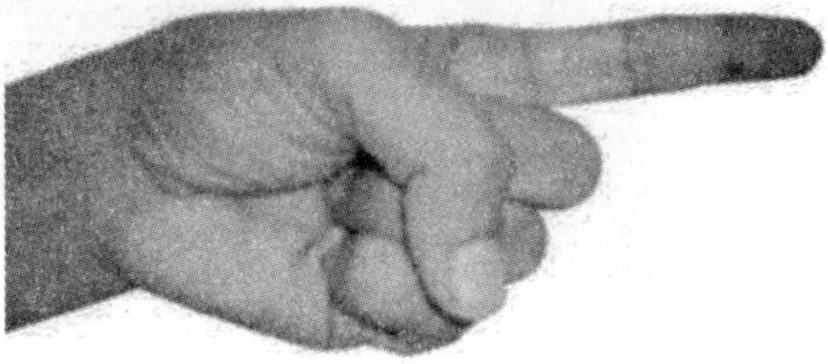

Index Finger

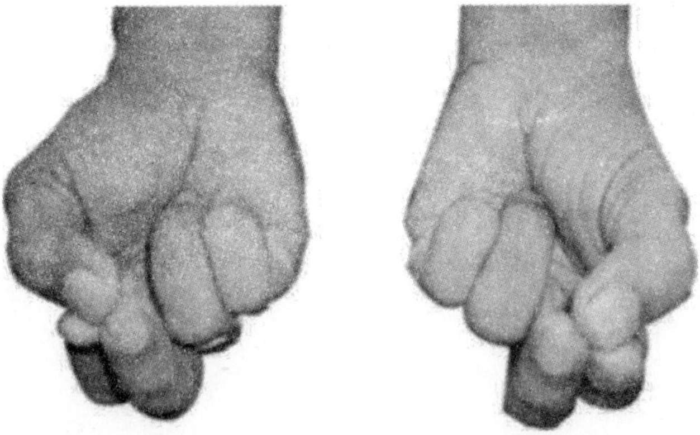

Kuber Mudra - for abundance

## Acknowledgments

1. Vedas, Upanishads, Six systems of Indian philosophy and Geeta. Literatures of: - Osho and Swami Satyanand Sarasvati, Bihar School of Yoga Munger Bihar.

Reiki - Master Mikao Usui (The Founder), Paula Horan, Walter Luback, Robert Lee Rand, Thorson.

Master Choa Kok Sui.


**Popular is not always right and right is rarely popular.**

**Excellence is rarely found and even more rarely valued.**

**Seek complete freedom.**

**"There is life beyond the stars.**

**There is life that knows no bars."**

## About The Author

Born in Karachi (Pakistan) on 12-09-1939 and migrated to India in 1947 along with his parents during the partition of the country. After Master's Degree in Sanskrit from D.A.V. College Jalandhar, he joined teaching profession. Two years later, to quench his spiritual thirst, he became a preacher in Arya Samaj and there after he devoted his whole life in spiritual studies and meditations. Formerly he was a poet in Hindi, Sanskrit and English and a gazal - writer. As a writer his journey began from Hello! (A booklet published in 1990) to The Healing Hands.

He is a consultant and exponent of Reiki - Healing, Chakra meditations, Breath - Balancing, Basic pranic - healing, meditations of Osho, Raj Yoga and mudras. His ideal is -

**"Enjoy the effort, if aim is good,**

**To the result, pay not heed.**

**You may not be understood**

**But blessed is your deed".**

**-The Publisher**

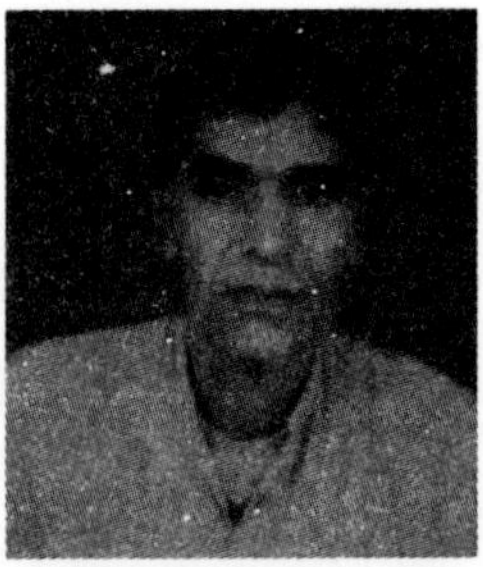

**Swami Nigmanand Sarasvati**

Ph: 87900 60291

Gauri Ashram, Bahadur pally

Hyderabad, A.P. Pin - 500043